I0424305

I Beat Heart Disease,
So Can You

The graphic drawing has been done by K.B. Graphics Co. in East Rochester, NY

I Beat Heart Disease, So Can You

Guido V. Marinetti, Ph.D.

iUniverse, Inc.
New York Lincoln Shanghai

I Beat Heart Disease, So Can You

Copyright © 2006 by Guido V. Marinetti

All rights reserved. No part of this book may be used or reproduced by any means, graphic, electronic, or mechanical, including photocopying, recording, taping or by any information storage retrieval system without the written permission of the publisher except in the case of brief quotations embodied in critical articles and reviews.

iUniverse books may be ordered through booksellers or by contacting:

iUniverse
2021 Pine Lake Road, Suite 100
Lincoln, NE 68512
www.iuniverse.com
1-800-Authors (1-800-288-4677)

Permission has been granted free of charge to use information in my previous book "Disorders of Lipid Metabolism" published by Plenum Press in 1990 on the following condition: full credit (book, journal, title, volume, year of publication, page, chapter/article title, name(s) of author(s), figure number, original copyright notice) is given to the publication in which the material was originally published by adding: With kind permission of Springer Science and Business Media.

Permission has been granted by Mr. Brad Lemley to use material in his article "What Does Science Say We Should Eat" that was published in Discover Magazine, February 2006, pages 43–49.

ISBN-13: 978-0-595-39580-4 (pbk)
ISBN-13: 978-0-595-83983-4 (ebk)
ISBN-10: 0-595-39580-5 (pbk)
ISBN-10: 0-595-83983-5 (ebk)

Printed in the United States of America

Eat to live or eat to die
Too much of a "good" thing can kill you

Contents

List of Illustrations (Figures)

Tables

Preface

Heart disease and stroke are two leading causes of death in the United States and the world. Elevated blood lipids (fats) especially cholesterol and triglycerides cause atherosclerosis that predisposes persons to heart disease and stroke. Unfortunately these diseases begin early in life and continue slowly over the life span of affected individuals. Diet, genes, stress, and environment play an important role in the etiology and treatment of heart disease.

Moreover, diets high in refined carbohydrates have caused an epidemic of obesity in the U.S. I have included a chapter that explains how excess carbohydrate is converted to glucose that then is converted to excess fat and causes obesity and diabetes. The latter are risk factors for coronary artery disease (CAD). Fortunately this disease is treatable and curable by diets, exercise, and lipid lowering drugs.

My personal experience with heart disease and my education as a professor of Biochemistry at a major U.S. medical school provide my credentials to write this book. I have taught medical students how lipids are metabolized, how high levels of blood lipids cause atherosclerosis and heart disease, and how these diseases are treated by diets, exercise, and drugs.

Many books have been written on diets and cholesterol but they do not cover adequately the science behind these health problems. My book provides some of the science background of blood lipids, heart disease, diet, and drug therapies for lowering blood lipids (cholesterol and triglycerides). In order to understand topics such as saturated and polyunsaturated fatty acids, obesity, blood lipoproteins, cholesterol, HDL, LDL, triglycerides, omega-3 fatty acids, the metabolic syndrome, atherosclerosis, statin drugs, and how diets and drugs work to lower blood lipids the public needs more basic science information on the these critical health topics.

I have divided the book into three parts in order to satisfy the varied educational backgrounds of the potential readers of my book.

Part 1 has some background of my life and how I beat coronary heart disease. Part 1 also has an Introduction that covers some elementary aspects of biochemistry and the types of lipids. This part may be optional reading for some readers and is done to prepare the readers for the next sections of the book.

Part 2 has chapters 1 through 4 that cover the main topics, including digestion of foods, diet and drug treatments for high levels of blood lipids, and the history of atherosclerosis. Part 2 provides information on how persons can use diets, drugs, and exercise to win the battle of heart disease. The benefits of knowing which types of carbohydrates, proteins, and fish omega-3 fatty acids to eat are vital to prevent or protect oneself from heart disease and cancer.

Part 3 covers the science (biochemistry) of the metabolism of fatty acids, cholesterol, blood lipoproteins, and how excess dietary glucose is converted to fat. The readers choose which parts of the book are more important and of more interest to them. To be better informed on this important health topic I recommend reading all three parts of the book. Learning a bit of science can be enjoyable, helpful and a rewarding challenge.

Cholesterol is often branded as a "bad" molecule because it is associated with plaques in arteries. But all the cells of our body need enough cholesterol to make cell membranes, steroid hormones and vitamin D. Furthermore, too little cholesterol may be harmful to good health. The human body makes all the cholesterol it needs. However, excess dietary cholesterol, excess dietary saturated and trans fats, and excess dietary carbohydrates, lead to high levels of blood cholesterol and triglycerides that over time cause atherosclerosis and heart disease.

Two other features of this book are how obesity, the metabolic syndrome, and drinking alcohol in excess affect blood lipids and the heart. These topics are not well covered in most books on diets. Yet excess alcohol consumption, obesity, and the metabolic syndrome continue to be major health and economic problems in the U.S.

Information is a very important commodity in today's world. The more the public knows about the very elementary science of diets, drugs, and heart disease the better they can take care of their health and the better they will understand how diets and drugs work and how they help in treating and preventing heart disease and extending ones lifespan.

In this book I shall use the word blood, rather than plasma, when referring to the laboratory values of lipids. Plasma is the supernatant fluid obtained when whole blood is centrifuged (spun). Serum is the supernatant fluid obtained when whole blood is allowed to clot and then is centrifuged. Analysis of blood lipids is normally done on plasma. Also the terms such as LDL, HDL, VLDL, and IDL referring to lipoproteins in blood denote the plural tense. Thus LDL refers to low density lipoproteins (not lipoprotein).

Acknowledgement

I thank my daughter Hope and son Tim for their help in preparing the tables of this book, for formatting the manuscript, and for suggestions on altering the book. I dedicate this book to my family and to the general public. Special thanks to my wife Antoinette for her patience and support during the long time required to write this book.

List of Abbreviations

A, adenine, a nitrogen base found in DNA

ACTH, adrenocorticotropic hormone

ADH, alcohol dehydrogenase, an enzyme which oxidizes alcohol

ADP, adenosine diphosphate, a precursor to ATP

ALDH, aldehyde dehydrogenase, another enzyme which oxidizes alcohol

α, the Greek symbol alpha

AMP, adenosine monophosphate

cAMP, cyclic adenosine monophosphate, a second messenger molecule in cells

ATP, adenosine triphosphate, the chemical storage form of energy in our body

β, the Greek symbol beta

BMI, body mass index used to calculate obesity

C, cytosine a base in DNA

C-9, carbon atom 9 in fatty acids

CAD, coronary artery disease

CAT-I, carnitine acylCoA transferase-I, an enzyme involved in fatty acid metabolism

CAT-II, carnitine acylCoA transferase-II, same as CAT-I-

CETP, cholesterol ester transfer protein, transfers cholesterol among blood lipoproteins

cDNA, copy deoxyribonucleic acid

CHD, coronary heart disease

CE, cholesterol ester, cholesterol containing a fatty acid in an ester bond

Chol, cholesterol, a major and important lipid in blood and in cell membranes cm, centimeter

CNS, central nervous system consisting of the spinal cord and the brain

CO_2 carbon dioxide a gas formed by oxidation of foods

CoA, coenzyme A, an important substrate in the metabolism of fats and glucose

COX-I, cyclooxygenase I, a constitutive enzyme that converts polyunsaturated fatty acids to prostaglandins

COX-II, cyclooxygenase-II, an inducible enzyme that converts polyunsaturated fatty acids to prostaglandins

DHA, docosahexenoic acid, has 20 carbon atoms and 4 double bonds and is a n-3 type fatty acid

dl deciliter. One tenth of a liter

DNA, deoxyribonucleic acid, the genetic substance of all living cells, contains deoxyglucose and the nitrogen bases A, T, G, and C

EPA, eicosapentenoic acid, a fatty acids with 20 carbon atoms and 5 double bonds, is an n-3 fatty acid and is found mainly in fish

FA, fatty acids are lipid molecules found in all living cells. They vary in chain length and in the number of double bonds.

g gram

g/g gram per gram

GLUT, glucose transport protein, an important protein involved in glucose entry and exit from cells

GTP, guanosine triphosphate

H^+ hydrogen atom or proton

HDL, high density lipoprotein, carries excess cholesterol from other organs to the liver

HL, hepatic lipase, an enzyme which degrades the lipids of chylomicron remnants in the liver

HMGCoA, hydroxymethylglutaryl-CoA, the important intermediate in cholesterol synthesis

HMGR, hydroxymethylglutarylCoA reductase, the regulatory enzyme in the synthesis of cholesterol and which is inhibited by the Statin drugs

H_2O, water

IDDM, insulin dependent diabetes

IDL, intermediate density lipoprotein that carries cholesterol in the blood

Kcal, kilocalorie, equal to 1000 calories

Kg, kilogram, equal to 1000 grams

LDL, low density lipoprotein, the main carrier of cholesterol in the blood, high levels may cause heart disease, often called bad cholesterol

LOX, lipooxygease, an enzyme that oxidizes polyunsaturated fatty acids that often are inflammatory in the body

LP, lipoprotein, carries lipids in the blood

LPL, lipoprotein lipase, the main enzyme which degrades blood lipoproteins

mg, milligram, one thousandth of a gram

MCT, medium chain triglycerides, contain short chain fatty acids and are used in diets to treat persons having very high levels of blood triglycerides

mRNA, messenger ribonucleic acid, carries the genetic information from DNA to make proteins

NAD, nicotinamide adenine dinucleotide (oxidized form) a vitamin coenzyme

NADH, nicotinamide adenine dinucleotide (reduced form), a vitamin coenzyme

NSAID, non-steroidal anti-inflammatory drugs such as aspirin, ibuprofen, Alleve, Advil and Celebrex

NEFA, non esterified fatty acid, free fatty acids in the blood.

NIDDM, non-insulin dependent diabetes

nm, nanometer, one billionth of a meter

PE, phosphatidylethanolamine, a type of phospholipid found in cell membranes

PC, phosphatidlycholine, a type of phospholipid found in cell membranes

PDGF, platelet derived growth factor, a protein factor which stimulates the synthesis of smooth muscle cells in arteries

Pi, inorganic phosphate

PL, phospholipid, a generic name for lipids having a phosphate group

PS, phosphatidylserine, a phospholipid found in cell membranes

PUFA, polyunsaturated fatty acids that contain two or more double bonds

RDA, required daily requirement (usually of vitamins)

RNA, ribonucleic acid, comes in several forms that contain the nitrogen bases A, U, G, and C and the sugar ribose, and are involved in protein synthesis

SRE, sterol regulatory element, involved in the regulation of gene activity

SREBP, sterol regulatory element binding protein, a protein which binds to and controls the activity of SRE

T thymine, a nitrogen base found in DNA

TG, triglyceride, a lipid containing three fatty acids linked to glycerol and is the storage form of energy in fat cells

TXA, thromboxane, a prostaglandin that causes blood platelets to aggregate and form a clot

U, uracil, a nitrogen base found in RNA

U.S., United States

VLDL, very low density lipoprotein, blood lipoproteins that transport mainly triglycerides

> designates greater than

< designates less than

WHL waist to hip ratio

Part 1

Chronology and Introduction

Chronology

Background of My Life

When I was a young boy I enjoyed outdoor life and was fortunate to live next to woods and ponds, where I would search for frogs, garter snakes, and salamanders. I also imagined that I was a frontiersman searching for turkeys and Indians in the woods and was disappointed when I found none.

I and other young boys in the neighborhood organized a baseball team. We played other teams in our area. Without the necessary funds, we could not afford uniforms and got used balls and bats from the older boy's teams. During my college years I was a pitcher on the graduate student's baseball team. We played for fun and had no uniforms and played against the four medical student teams and other graduate student teams. I pitched and won the last deciding game against the medical students. As I grew older I continued my interest in sports and played tennis and golf.

During summer months when I was in grammar school, I and other young boys and girls in the neighborhood worked on farms picking vegetables and fruits. The farmer would pick us up early in the morning in his big truck and then take us home later in the afternoon. It was hard sweaty work but the money came in handy.

I also enjoyed reading books. Two books had a big influence on my later life. *Microbe Hunters by Paul de Kruif* was the first book and *Arrowsmith by Sinclair Lewis* was the second book. The first book fascinated me by the manner in which scientists discovered bacteria and how they worked to kill the harmful ones. The second book gave me insight into how doctors do research and give their lives to treat ill patients under difficult circumstances.

I was selected to be standard bearer in the 8th grade of grammar school. My home room teacher told me to report to the principal. I wondered what was going on. What did I do wrong? When I got to her office my fears were relieved when she told me I was selected to be the standard bearer because of my good grades. I had no idea what a standard bearer was and what it meant for me. It turned out to be an honor. However I had to raise and lower the U.S.

flag every school day. This meant getting up early in the morning and staying a bit later after school.

After grammar school I was transferred to high school. Grammar school was near my house but high school was quite far away. I and other students walked 3 miles one way to high school regardless of the weather. There were no school buses at this time. During cold winter days and very rainy days walking 6 miles round trip was not very pleasant. One very cold winter day, when the weather was close to 30 degrees below zero, my eye lids and nose became so caked with ice that I had a hard time finding my way. Fortunately this did not happen too often.

The students from poor families brought their own lunches and ate them in the hallways during cold or wet weather. Students from well-off families ate their lunches in the school cafeteria. I came from a poor family and never had my lunch in the cafeteria. During summer months eating our lunches outside was fun.

I desperately wanted to go to college but my parents could not afford it. A job after high school was hard to find. World War II came and I was drafted into the U. S. Army. I had basic training for three months in Utah during the cold months of January through March. This meant many hours of marching, drilling, and going through a very difficult obstacle course. The training put me in excellent physical condition and I felt great. During this training time several soldiers and I had to sleep in a large tent that had a central coal heated stove. We took turns to watch and feed stove during the night. One night a heavy snow accumulated on the tent and the tent collapsed. We were fortunate that the tent did not burn from the hot stove.

Later in the spring the camp was hit with a strong sand storm that lasted for several days. Sand was in our barracks, in our beds, in our clothes, and in our food. This now made me appreciate what the current U.S. soldiers are facing in Iraq. We had to continue drilling each day during the snow and sand storms. As a result of sand storm, half of the soldiers in the camp came down with respirator infections. The Army base commander was changed after this fiasco.

I was happy when the training ended and was sent to an Army X-Ray school in Denver. This school trained a select group of soldiers to dismantle and reassemble a mobile X-ray machine to be used in a field hospital. Later, I was transferred to the *U.S. Air Force Tactical Air Center* in Orlando, Florida where I worked in the military hospital as an X-ray technician for a few months.

Later I was selected to work in a laboratory of the *United States Department of Agriculture* in Orlando, Florida. The head of the laboratory sent me to

Atlanta GA to special school to learn how to dissect mosquitoes and identify the malaria parasites.

The laboratory consisted of a group of soldiers from the *United States Tactical Air Force Base* and a group of scientists from the *U.S. Department of Agriculture.* The laboratory was under the supervision of *U.S. Air Force* General H. Arnold. It had the urgent and high priority job of protecting the troops from getting malaria and other insect borne diseases in the south Pacific war zone. The laboratory had three major goals. One was to find and then develop methods for impregnating the uniforms with safe insecticides that would kill the mosquitoes that carried the malaria parasite. The second was to develop repellents in the form of creams to put on the skin. The third was to develop sprays for spaying the jungle areas around the troops.

Many hundreds of chemicals were tested. I recall vividly the day that DDT was found to be a very potent killer of mosquitoes. A loud shout went through lab. At about the same time the British scientists discovered a compound that they labeled 666. Many pounds of DDT were ordered and placed outside of the lab. Unfortunately, the toxicity of DDT was not known. The very large amounts of DDT were needed to make large volumes low concentrations of DDT that were tested by spraying over the jungle areas in Florida.

Some of the soldiers including myself volunteered as subjects for the insect repellents put on the skin of each subject. Some soldiers served as controls (no active repellent) and other soldiers had the repellents. No one knew which one he had. We had to go into the jungle areas for several hours and then go back to the lab to find out how many mosquito bites each one had. Fortunately I had only a very few bites but other soldiers had many bites that were irritating and painful.

The laboratory was getting ready to move to the South Pacific but this did not happen because the war ended when the atomic bombs were dropped on Japan. I was informed by the head of the laboratory that I was chosen to work in the laboratory because of my work at a biological company back home and because of my good score on the Army intelligent test. Whatever the reasons were, I was delighted to have this unique opportunity to work in the laboratory.

This research was very successful. After the war, estimates are that by preventing mosquito bites it prevented malaria and saved the lives of thousands of the U.S. troops in the Pacific war zone. Each person in the laboratory was given the Distinguished Service Award by Clinton Anderson, *U.S. Secretary of the Department of Agriculture.*

I wondered later if any of the personnel and soldiers developed serious health effects from exposure to DDT. It does not appear to have had any serious effect on my health. Years later after the war many birds in Florida were found to have died from DDT poisoning and DDT was removed from the market even though during and after the war it saved the lives of many thousands of people living in India, Asia, Africa, and the Pacific Islands.

My military experience had a major effect of my life. I was determined to get higher education and become a scientist. It renewed my interest in science when I was a young boy. The G. I. Bill of Rights offered returning soldiers a once in a life-time chance to go to college. I and many other soldiers took advantage of this great offer that paid for most of our college education. Biochemistry appealed to me because it dealt with the chemistry of life. I wanted to learn how living cells function at the molecular level.

To do this I needed a higher graduate education. I first earned a B.S. degree in Chemistry and later got a Ph.D. degree in Biochemistry. After twelve years of teaching and doing research I was promoted to full professor at the *University Of Rochester Medical School.* My responsibilities at the *University of Rochester Medical School* were to teach medical students and graduate students and to do research.

My teaching area covered the structure, metabolism, and function of lipids, the role of lipids in atherosclerosis and heart disease, and the function of lipids in cell membranes. My research also dealt with developing methods for separating and analyzing phospholipids, the biosynthesis of phospholipids, and measuring membrane hormone receptors for insulin and epinephrine. This research was among the first to show that fat cells from obese patients had less insulin receptors than fat cells from non-obese patients. Persons with less insulin receptors cannot metabolize fats and sugars as well as persons that have the normal number of insulin receptors.

In the mid 1980s I teamed up with two clinicians, Dr. Gilbert Forbes and Dr. Robert Campbell, to initiate one of the first organized courses in nutrition for first year medical students at the *University of Rochester.* We named the course *"The Biochemistry of Nutrition."* This course stimulated other medical schools to start similar courses in nutrition since it became apparent that nutrition was very important in preventive medicine.

Drs. Forbes, Campbell and I realized that in the 1980s there was much misunderstanding on diets and their role in heart disease. The 1980s was a period of high interest in diets as related to heart disease but there was much lack of information on the types of lipids, especially the types of saturated and polyunsaturated fatty acids (n-3 versus n-6) and much conflict on which diets were the best. The nutrition course we started was aimed to clarify these issues and also covered the nutritional aspects of the metabolism of lipids, proteins, and carbohydrates.

Dietary fats acquired a bad name in the mid 1980s. *The American Heart Association* recommended that the public decrease the daily fat intake to thirty percent or less of total calories. This was done without appreciating the importance of the different types of saturated and polyunsaturated fatty acids. Low fat diets were recommended in spite of the fact that people living in the Mediterranean area were known to consume a lot of olive oil and have less heart disease than Americans. These people also work harder outdoors than most Americans. Unfortunately most Americans began to eat more carbohydrates to get enough food calories. This turned out to be a disaster because it led to a high increase in body weight, obesity, and type-2 diabetes and increased the risk of heart disease.

We informed medical students that increasing dietary carbohydrates was not a good thing. As a biochemist, I knew that excess carbohydrate is converted to glucose, which the human body converts to fat. I also informed the students about the different types of fatty acids especially the n-3 (omega-3) fatty acids which occur in high amount in fish and suggested that they eat more fish, less carbohydrate, and exercise daily.

During the 1980s, the public also was advised to avoid eating eggs because they contain a high level of cholesterol in the yolk (about 300 mg per yolk). However, nothing was said about the "good" phospholipids found in egg yolk. I followed the advice and avoided eating eggs even though there were no compelling studies which showed that eating several eggs a week was harmful. It shows how fear can make a person believe unreasonable information.

The faculty decided to have all the first year medical students get their blood lipids analyzed by the hospital clinical blood laboratory. We discussed the results of these tests. I also trained the medical students how to analyze their own blood cholesterol. Some students were surprised to find that they had high levels of blood cholesterol or triglycerides and they immediately were concerned and asked for more information on what type of diets or drugs they should begin taking.

Later when we questioned the students about their family background we found that several of these students had a parent, aunt, or uncle who had heart disease. These students learned a good lesson by starting early on diets and exercise to lower their high levels of blood lipids. This information has enhanced their chance of avoiding heart disease. Some of these students had a hard time believing that high levels of blood cholesterol could happen to them since they were young. Medical students also learned how their future patients would feel when they had to give a blood sample and more so the apprehension when waiting for the results of the tests. Our hope was that their experience made them better doctors.

Another major health problem occurred in the 1980s when food producers began to hydrogenate the vegetable oils that were used to make margarines as a substitute for butter. Butter has a higher content of saturated fat than margarine. This advice led to unfavorable results because the process of partial hydrogenation used to make margarines, converted the natural unsaturated fatty acids in the vegetable oils to trans fatty acids. Later trans fatty acids were found to be a high risk factor for heart disease.

Indeed trans fats were more of a risk that saturated fats. This meant that eating the hydrogenated margarines was worse than eating butter and much worse than eating the natural vegetable oils. Having a chemistry background I knew that partial hydrogenation of fatty acids altered the double bonds of the natural polyunsaturated fatty acids because I used hydrogenation of lipids in my research.

During this time, Dr. Atkins wrote a diet book that had a radical idea. He recommended a diet high in proteins and high in fat but low in carbohydrates. How could this diet make sense when the American Heart Institute was advising the public to eat less fat? The Atkins diet did make persons lose weight. However, the very high protein diet was not good for persons with kidney disease and also increased the risk to some persons (especially diabetic persons) of getting ketosis (the accumulation of certain organic ketoacids) from the high amount of fat in the diet. Some persons also were at risk of developing an imbalance of potassium in the body that might adversely affect heart rhythm

Many books soon came out on diets. Some like the Ornish diet and later the Willett diet were reasonable and based on sound science. Some diets, such as the diet based on blood types, and the diet based on eating proteins, carbohydrate and fats on alternate days were not based on sound science. Dr. Willett has made similar points on the past history of diets and the mistakes that were made by the *American Heart Association* and other scientists during the 1980s. The effects of diets on blood lipids and heart disease are covered in Chapter 2.

How I Beat Coronary Artery Disease (CAD)

I write this section for those who may develop coronary artery disease with the hope that they may learn from my experience. First I point out that thousands of men and women have had open heart surgery for coronary artery disease. However, for each individual the outcome and experience differs.

I did not expect what was to happen in my life. In January of 1980 I was a visiting Professor at the University of Arizona in Tucson, One cool wet day I experienced chest discomfort when jogging and later when playing tennis. I also experienced a pain in my left jaw. The pain radiated down to my little left finger. I knew immediately that these were symptoms of a heart problem. I never smoked, always had a normal weight, but tried to convince myself that this could not happen to me. I had to consider that I may have inherited a genetic predisposition to heart disease. This later on proved to be true.

As soon as I returned home in April of 1980 I saw my doctor. He took a blood sample to check my blood lipids. To my surprise my blood cholesterol level was 320 mg/dl and my triglyceride level was 250 mg/dl. These are abnormally high values. How could this happen to me.? The normal value for cholesterol should be below 200 mg/dl and the normal value for triglycerides should be below 150 mg/dl. In 1980 the field of cholesterol and diets was new and little information was known on what were normal values of blood lipids. Indeed, a cholesterol value of 300 mg/dl was not considered very high. There was much conflict on how to treat patients and the Statin drugs had not yet been developed.

I did not pass a stress test. The electrocardiograms taken during the test indicated that one or more of my coronary arteries may be occluded with lipid plaque. To check this I was given an angiogram. The angiogram is done by inserting a catheter into the large femoral artery in the groin and slowly working the artery up and past the arch of the aortic artery in order to have access to the openings of the coronary arteries. Radio-opaque dye is then injected into the right and left main coronary arteries and a series of X-rays are taken to visualize the arteries to see how badly they are occluded. Both the right main and the left main coronary arteries were about 90 percent occluded with cholesterol plaques.

During the angiogram I felt some discomfort when the dye was injected. This lasts only a few seconds and goes away when the blood flow removes the dye. A sand bag is placed over the femoral artery where the catheter is inserted in order to stop the blood from leaking until the artery is healed. This healing may take several hours.

My doctor and I had to decide what to do next. The best choice in my case was open heart coronary artery bypass surgery. Stents were not well developed at this time. Because both two main coronary arteries were badly occluded and the left circumflex artery had a partial occlusion, the decision was made to perform open heart surgery and use veins in one leg as grafts to bypass the occluded coronary arteries.

In 1980 coronary artery bypass surgery was in the early stage of development. I asked the surgeon how many of these operations he had done and what was his track record. I was convinced he had performed enough of this type of surgery and 90 percent were successful. But one always has to consider the 10 percent of surgeries that have side effects.

There was a one to two percent chance that I might die from the operation but I had a ninety percent chance of a successful outcome. I found these to be favorable odds considering that if I did not have the surgery I would probably die within a few years with a massive heart attack. One often hears the advice "get your house in order" if one has an incurable disease. I did not have an incurable disease but I decided to get my house in order. I informed my wife and two children about my finances and preparation for a funeral and where to find the necessary information on insurance policies. This was not easy or pleasant for me and my family but it had to be done.

I had to wait two months for the surgery. The waiting had plenty of apprehensive moments and sleepless nights of worry. During this time I went on a low calorie diet to decrease my blood lipids but in retrospect, this was a mistake. For my height of five feet eleven inches, my weight of 158 lbs. was normal. The diet dropped my weight to 145 lbs. A person with my weight did not have to lose weight before surgery. Also, after major surgery most patients will lose weight and too much weight loss may make for a more difficult recovery time.

To perform the surgery the surgeon places the patient on a special heart-lung machine so that the blood flow from the heart is diverted to the machine, gets oxygenated, and gets back into the body. During this time the patient's body is cooled down and the heart stops beating. This allows the highly trained surgeon to open the chest cavity by cutting through the sternum. This opening of the chest allows access to the heart and for the surgeon to perform the operation. The surgeon has to sew the vein grafts on the base of the aorta and on the coronary arteries. They have to be careful that any valves in the veins open in the correct direction.

The surgery was successful but I developed a problem. I was put into the ICU (intensive care unit) the attending doctor found that blood was leaking from one of the vein grafts. I was not aware of this since I had not yet awakened from the surgery. My family told me that I was immediately taken back to surgery and the surgeon had to reopen my chest to find and stop the bleeding. I was put back in the ICU unit for 10 more days.

When I awoke from the surgery I was put on assisted breathing in the ICU. My recovery was long and painful because of the repeated surgery. I went home after 10 days and had a very tough recovery with pain, loss of appetite; and loss of interest in life. I was able to do some of my research planning at home after about 5 weeks of healing. I slowly recovered and after two and one half months went back to work. Today surgeons have gained greater skills and open heart by pass operations are done quicker and patients are usually released within one week after the operation.

After the surgery I went on a modest diet similar to the Willett diet, and was given the new drug Mevacor plus the drug Lopid. Mevacor was first statin drug of many other statins that were discovered later. Mevacor was used to lower the blood cholesterol level and Lopid was used to lower the blood triglyceride level. Unfortunately during the mid 1980's the statin drugs were new and little was known about their side effects and how they would interact with other drugs…

Later studies showed that the combination of Mevacor and Lopid was a very bad one because it gave me severe muscle pains. I realized that something was wrong and stopped the Lopid. Several years later when more patients were put on these drugs some patients developed severe muscle pains and a few developed a condition called rhabdomyolysis. This latter condition can lead to kidney damage and death. Fortunately, only a very few patients get rhabdomyolysis and die. Today the use of a Statin drug with either Lopid or Niacin has been stopped.

Later more statin drugs were developed and I switched to Pravachol, then to Zocor and finally to Lipitor to lower my blood lipids. Lipitor is much superior to the early Mevacor. Lipitor treatment combined with a prudent diet was successful in normalizing my cholesterol level to 170 mg/dl, my triglycerides to below 150 mg/dl, and my LDL cholesterol to below 100 mg/dl. I also did exercise by walking, playing tennis and golfing which I continue to the present time. My weight has remained normal and I have managed to survive for many years after the surgery and lead a normal life. However without follow-up therapy with diet, statin drugs, and exercise, it is likely that I would not have survived these additional years. I thus was able to beat heart disease and others can do the same thing. Unfortunately my father did not have this new medical knowledge and died of a heart attack at age 72. Thus knowledge prolongs ones life span and allows one to live a normal healthy and happy life for a much longer time. Below I list the most important information and recommendations on how to beat heart disease.

The Most Important Points on How to Beat Heart Disease

1. Check your family genetic background.

2. Get your blood lipids analyzed early in life.

3. See your doctor on a regular basis.

4. Eat a balanced diet of vegetables, fruits, nuts, good proteins, good carbohydrates, and good fats. I use and recommend the Willett Diet. Avoid refined carbohydrates found in white rice, pasta, and potato, and sweets. Eat high fiber and high wheat pasta, high wheat breads, and unrefined brown rice. Eat poultry and fish in place of red meat and fatty steaks. Eat fish and vegetable oils high in omega-3 fatty acids. Refer to chapter 2.

5. The most beneficial dietary fatty acids are DHA and EPA that are found in fish. They provide protection against heart disease, stroke, cancer, inflammation and blood clots. Refer to chapters 2 and 3.

5. Exercise daily by walking at least 30 minutes each day or walking three times a day for 10 minutes. The use of treadmills or bicycle type equipment is good for those who can afford to buy these. In very cold or very hot weather walk in malls or do exercises in your home Refer to chapter 3...

6. Those who have had or who are at high risk for coronary artery disease should look into taking dietary supplements such as folic acid, aspirin, L-carnitine or L-acetylcarnitine, alpha lipoic acid, and fish oil omega-3 fatty acids capsules on a daily basis or three to four times a week. Refer to chapter 3.

7. Those who have high levels of blood cholesterol and/or triglycerides should first go on diets for three to six months to lower their blood lipids before taking lipid-lowering drugs. Use drugs only if diets do not lower your blood lipids enough. Refer to chapters 2 and 3.

8. For those who have high levels of blood cholesterol, the most effective drugs are the Statins (such as Lipitor, Zocor, Pravachol, Crestor, and Vytorin). Start on the lowest dose and increase the dose if needed. Refer to chapter 3.

9. Those with high levels of triglycerides can take the drugs Niacin or Lopid. Refer to chapter 3.

10. Persons that have high levels of both blood cholesterol and triglycerides may take Lipitor plus Colestid or Lipitor plus a plant sterol. Or they can take Vytorin that contains both a statin and a synthetic sterol. Vegetables contain plant sterols so that eating more vegetables may substitute in part for drugs containing plant sterols Refer to chapter 3.

11. The goal is to keep the total blood cholesterol level below 200 mg/dl, the LDL cholesterol level below 100 mg/dl, the HDL cholesterol level above 40 mg/dl and the blood triglyceride level below 130 mg/dl. Refer to chapters 6 and 7.

12. Persons that have high cholesterol levels should not eat more than four whole eggs a week or may eat egg white and avoid eating fatty steaks, liver, and kidney.

13. Avoid stress as much as is possible. Prolonged stress may cause hormone imbalance in the body and some researchers believe may influence adversely the body metabolism that is regulated by the brain.

14. Avoid overeating and smoking, and check your blood pressure on a routine basis.

15. If you have symptoms of a heart attack such as chest pain or tightness, pain radiating from your lower left teeth to the left finger or fingers, shortness of breath, nausea, sweating or feel like fainting, call 911 immediately and take one 325 mg aspirin pill.

16. Eating should be enjoyable. Eat slowly, savor the taste and avoid distractions. Occasionally, but not too often, it is ok to have a fatty steak or some type of dessert.

Introduction to General Concepts of Biochemistry and Types of Lipids

I have included this Introduction to give readers the background to appreciate the science behind diets and drug therapies for the treatment of heart disease and to understand better the chapters that follow.

All living cells carry out thousands of chemical reactions in an organize manner. Living cells contain lipids, proteins, carbohydrates, nucleic acids, vitamins, and minerals and water. Indeed, cells contain about 70 percent water. Since lipids are not soluble in water, they are combined with proteins to make lipoproteins which are more soluble Also, lipids were made very early in the evolution of living cells.

Cell membranes are essential for living organisms since they form an external coating of the cell to keep the internal parts from leaking into the environment. Membranes also divide the cells into internal domains and compartmentalize the many chemical reactions that occur in each cell. Membranes control the flow of nutrients, ions, waste products, and water in and out of cells. Membranes contain receptor proteins that react with hormones and drugs and also allow for the transmission of electrochemical nerve impulses in peripheral nerves and in the brain.

Lipids are essential for life and have an important role in medicine and in disease. The most important lipid related diseases are cardiovascular disease, obesity, diabetes, and cancer.

Biochemistry literally means the chemistry of life. All living cells are like little chemical factories that simultaneously carry out thousands of reactions. The term metabolism is the sum of all the chemical reactions that occur in the body. Anabolism refers to those reactions that make the essential chemicals in the cell, including proteins, lipids, carbohydrates, and nucleic acids. These reactions require energy. Catabolism refers to the breakdown of proteins, lipids, carbohydrates, and nucleic acids. This process produces energy some of which is heat and some is in the form of high energy chemicals such as ATP (adenosinetriphosphate).

The chemical reactions of living cells require protein catalysts called enzymes. All proteins are made from small molecules called amino acids. These are linked together in a linear array by a chemical bond called the peptide bond that forms products called polypeptides. The linear polypeptides then arrange themselves in a complex three dimension structure that is the finished protein.

Some proteins such as collagen, serve as structural components of cells. Other proteins serve as enzymes that catalyze the chemical reactions that either build up or degrade other molecules. Enzymes allow the reactions to occur at a rapid rate at the relatively low temperature of the body of 98.6 degrees F or 37 degrees C. Some enzymes require metal ions (calcium, magnesium, manganese, iron, zinc, etc) or coenzymes to function. Vitamins are essential for life and they act as coenzymes.

Enzymes are flexible three dimensional molecules which bind their substrates (the compounds they act on) in a very specific manner called the lock and key fit. The binding is aided by the ability of enzymes to change slightly their shape and allow the enzyme binding site to fit on the substrate. This specificity of binding allows researchers and pharmaceutical companies to make or find drugs which are similar but not identical to the substrate. These drugs bind sufficiently at the catalytic site of the enzyme to block the binding of the substrate. This blocks the enzyme from acting. The stating drugs are an example. They bind to the enzyme which controls the synthesis of cholesterol and this inhibits the liver from making excess cholesterol and lowers the level of cholesterol in the blood.

The genes of all cells are found in DNA (deoxyribonucleic acid). DNA consists of a linear array of four chemical components (called nitrogen bases) abbreviated as A, T, G and C, that respectively stand for adenine, thymine, guanine, and cytosine. DNA also contains the sugar deoxyribose that with the nitrogen bases forms the nucleotide monomers abbreviated as (ATP, GTP, CTP, and TTP). These sugar containing monomers are linked together and form the double helix structure of DNA. The double helix occur s because A always binds to T and G always binds to C by hydrogen bonds.

Two well known Noble prize winning scientists named James Watson and Francis Crick discovered the double helical structure of DNA from its X-Ray diffraction pattern. DNA replicates itself every time a cell divides to make a new cell. Sometimes a mistake in the linear sequence can occur but cells have the ability to correct most of these errors. Some of these errors may be innocuous while others may be lethal.

DNA contains the genetic code that consists of three of these bases in a linear array. Several billions of these triad bases occur in the linear DNA. This allows for many billions of arrangements that make up all the various genes in the plant and animal kingdom. The sequence and number of genes allows for the diversity of living organisms. DNA in eukaryote cells (cells that contain a nucleus) combines with proteins to form chromosomes.

Much of the DNA structure has no known function and has been called junk DNA. However, there is much dispute of this idea. Some researchers now believe that some of this junk DNA consists of viral DNA and some may be nonfunctional redundant DNA that was carried over from the millions of years that man has evolved. Some of the viral DNAs are oncogenes (cancer forming genes).

DNA has the instructions for producing all the 30,000 to 50,000 proteins of each living cell. It does so by first acting as a template to make other complex molecules called messenger RNA (ribonucleic acid). Messenger RNA (mRNA) contains the nitrogen bases A, U, G, and C and the sugar ribose. The process of DNA making RNA is called transcription since the genetic information in DNA is transcribed to messenger RNA. Several types of RNA are made. The ones called mRNA contain the transcribed genetic codes that are used to make proteins. The mRNAs interact with complex structures in the cell called ribosomes. Ribosomes act like little protein factories.

The complex of mRNA with ribosomes produces the proteins of the body using activated amino acids. Twenty amino acids produce these proteins. Ten of these amino acids are called essential since the human body cannot make these amino acids. The amino acids are arranged in a linear fashion to form the complex proteins. The process of mRNA coding for proteins is called translation since the information in the genetic code in mRNA is translated to the sequence of amino acids in the proteins.

Hormones are made in special organs called glands. Hormones activate enzyme reactions and control the synthesis of enzymes by activating the genes which code for the enzymes. Some hormones like insulin, glucagon, and epinephrine act by binding to specific receptor proteins that occur on cell membranes. The binding activates the receptor that then activates one or more other enzymes in a cascade amplification process called signal transduction. Other hormones such as the steroid hormones and thyroxine act in the nucleus of the cell where they are believed to influence the genes which code for specific enzymes or specific proteins.

Hormones occur in very low concentration in cells (micromolar to the picomolar range). Other hormones stimulate the production second messenger molecules such as cAMP (cyclic adenosine monophosphate) that activate other enzymes. Some hormones act directly or indirectly on the genes of DNA to stimulate the production of mRNAs. Transcription factors are molecules that bind to specific regions on DNA to stimulate (or inhibit) these genes that make mRNA. Promoter regions in the DNA contain segments called sterol regulatory elements (SREs) Other proteins called sterol regulatory element binding proteins (SREBPs) bind to the SREs and regulate the activity of the genes. They act as switches to turn on or turn off the genes.

During the course of evolution genetic changes have occurred that have altered the sequence of the bases in the genetic code. These changes can be innocuous or they can lead to fatal genetic diseases. The cure for these diseases will be very difficult and the best hope lies in stem cell research.

Molecular biology deals with biology at the subcellular and the cellular molecular level. This area of Biochemistry studies the molecules in the cell especially how DNA and mRNA function in the process of making proteins. Organ Biochemistry considers the interactions between the various organs at the macro level including the liver, kidneys, heart, intestines, muscles, skin, brain, and the various glandular organs. The glandular organs produce hormones that regulate the metabolism of the body.

The foods we eat are first digested in the mouth, stomach, and small intestines. Digestion requires specific enzymes and is regulated by hormones. The pancreas makes the digestive enzymes and also produces the hormones insulin and glucagon. The digested products are absorbed into the blood and made available to the organs of the body. The liver is the first organ to receive the digested foods from the blood.

The major function the liver is to use the digested products to synthesize lipids, proteins, glycogen, bile acids, and other macromolecules; and to detoxify drugs. Some of the proteins, lipids, and glucose made in the liver are used by other organs. The liver makes and breaks down glycogen to form glucose during starvation but during feeding the liver converts glucose to glycogen. The liver makes phospholipids, triglycerides, and cholesterol and converts these to lipoproteins that enter the blood and transport them to other organs. The liver is the chemical factory of the body.

The kidneys remove waste products from the blood (urea, ammonia, excess sodium, etc) and reabsorb essential nutrients (glucose, amino acids, potassium, etc). The heart pumps blood to all parts of the body. The heart beats about 100,000 times a day during which it pumps about 4000 gallons of blood through 60,000 miles of blood vessels, including the capillaries. The lungs take in oxygen and remove water and carbon dioxide that are the end products of the oxidation of lipids and glucose by the body.

The bone marrow makes red cells and white cells. Red blood cells carry oxygen to the organs of the body and carry carbon dioxide to the lungs. A major function of white blood cells is to produce antibodies to fight infections and to kill bacteria and viruses.

The functions of the brain are self evident but very complex and not well understood because of the many thousands of inter connections between the billions of brain cells. The biochemistry of the brain depends on the many neurotransmitters that it produces. Many of the neurotransmitters function by opening or closing special pores that act as gates in cell membranes Specific gates open and close to control the flux of ions like sodium, potassium, and calcium that produce nerve impulses. The brain contains the pituitary gland, called the master gland of the body, because in controls the functions of other glands. The brain also contains the pineal gland that produces melatonin, a hormone that regulates daily rhythms of the body and may act like a biological clock.

The brain normally oxidizes glucose but during starvation the brain can oxidize fatty acids. The same applies to skeletal muscle, heart muscle and kidneys. It is of interest that the oxidation of fatty acids produces more energy and water than does the oxidation of glucose. During a marathon run, the skeletal muscles and heart muscles first oxidize glucose and later when the stores of glucose (in the form of a large polymer called glycogen) are depleted the muscles then oxidize fatty acids. The body stores much more energy as fatty acids (as triglycerides) than it stores glucose as glycogen.

When too many fatty acids are oxidized they form acidic products that are called ketoacids. The excess production of these ketoacids causes a condition called ketoacidosis in which the acidity of the blood decreases to a point that makes a person go into a coma. This condition often occurs in diabetics that do not control their blood sugar levels. On the other hand if the blood sugar level gets too low this causes hypoglycemia (low blood sugar) that also can cause fainting or a coma. If the blood level of ammonia increases too much it also can make a person go into a coma. The level of these body chemicals is critical to normal health.

All the metabolic processes in the body organs are regulated by hormones and molecules called transcription factors. Some of their actions are mediated by specific hormone receptors that stimulate or inhibit specific enzymes or by the turning on or turning off specific genes. The body also makes other hormone like compounds called eicosanoids that consist of prostaglandins, leukotrienes, and lipoxins. Eicosanoids are made from polyunsaturated fatty acids. They are made is many cells of the body and have profound biological effects on most of the organs in the body. The hormones and the eicosanoids are made and degraded in a controlled manner by on and off chemical switches.

The chemical reactions in the body are in a steady state. This means that the molecules of the body such as proteins, lipids, carbohydrates and nucleic acids are made and degraded in a constant controlled manner. Thus at any one time the concentration of these products will rise and fall depending on their rates of synthesis and degradation.

When a doctor orders blood tests the results represent values at one single time point. It is analogous to looking at a movie picture one frame at a time. The true picture of what is happening is determined by looking at all the frames or doing multiple blood tests over a certain time interval. The latter however, is not practical for blood analyses from an economic point. Some blood tests, such as measuring blood triglycerides, are done on fasting blood. Unlike cholesterol whose level in the blood is fairly steady, triglyceride levels vary widely depending on how much fat is in the diet and if the person has consumed alcohol prior to the test.

In reality the body chemistry is in a continuous state of flux and the atoms in our body are constantly changing with time. But because the turnover of the body metabolism is so faithfully carried out we appear to look the same except for aging. We also are exchanging atoms with the persons, animals, and vegetation in our environment. This occurs with the carbon dioxide we breathe in and out and with the food we eat. The body uses the inhaled carbon dioxide to make certain chemicals. Trees use carbon dioxide for photosynthesis during the day and release oxygen during the night. We breathe in this carbon dioxide and oxygen and thus we exchange these atoms with our environment.

The exchange of atoms applies for the animal and plant foods we consume. However, the major difference is how the atoms are arranged in the proteins, fats, carbohydrates, and nucleic acids in the body. We are all a part of nature and share each others atoms. However, the instructions in DNA precisely dictate how these atoms are arranged in three dimension space. This makes every person a unique individual.

Types of Lipids

An introduction to the types of lipids that occur in the human body is helpful in appreciating the different types of lipids which occur in our bodies. Some lipids are used as fuel for energy production, some are essential for life, some are needed to make phospholipids for cell membranes, and some are substrates for the eicosanoids. The types of lipids are shown in the table below in Table 1.

Introduction Table 1. Types of lipids

Neutral Glycerol Lipids and Sterols:

Triglycerides, diglycerides, monoglycerides, (also called triacyl-glycerols, diacylglycerols, and monoacylglycerols).

Sterols—cholesterol, steroid hormones,

Fatty acids: saturated, monounsaturated, polyunsaturated types differ in chain length and in the number of double bonds.

Fatty acid derivatives having hormone like properties: the eicosanoids that include the leukotrienes, prostaglandins, and lipoxins.

Bile acids:

Cholic acid, deoxycholic acid, lithocholic acid, and chenodeoxy-cholic acid.

Glycerophospholipids:

Phosphatidylcholine, phosphatidylethanolamine, phosphatidylser-ine, phosphatidyinositols, phosphatidylglycerol, and cardiolipin.

Sphingolipids:

Sphingomyelin, ceramide, sphingosine-1-phosphate,

Glycosphingolipids:cerebrosides, sulfatides, gangliosides

Plasma lipoproteins

Chylomicrons, VLDL, IDL, LDL, HDL

NEFA—non esterified fatty acids bound to albumin

Some lipids have simple structures but others are very complex. This book will cover the triglycerides, fatty acids, cholesterol, and lipoproteins.

Lipids are essential components of all living cells. Phospholipids, sphingolipids, and cholesterol, make of the lipid bilayer structure of cell membranes. The membranes compartmentalize the cell into discrete domains, namely the nucleus, mitochondria, Golgi, endoplasmic reticulum, and peroxisomes. This allows the many thousands of chemical reactions in every cell to proceed in a very ordered way.

Most lipids are oily and not very soluble or very insoluble in water. Yet they occur in living cells that are made up of about 70 to 90 percent water. The lipids in the human body are associated with proteins to form lipoproteins that are more soluble in water and therefore more easily handled by the body.

Fatty acids are important fuels for living cells. Fatty acids are stored as triglycerides that are the main storage of chemical energy in cells. Eicosanoids are derived from the polyunsaturated fatty acids. Eicosanoids have hormone-like properties and are involved in inflammatory events in the body as well as in the regulation of the body organs. Bile acids are necessary for the digestion of dietary fats.

Fatty acids and other lipids play a vital role in medicine. The most important lipid related diseases are cardiovascular disease, obesity, diabetes, and cancer. Below in Table 2 are listed some of the major fatty acids of animal and plant cells.

Introduction Table 2. Major fatty acids of animals and plants *			
Fatty Acid Name	**No. of Carbon Atoms**	**No. of Double Bonds**	**Source**
Palmitic Acid	16	0	animal, plants
Stearic Acid	18	0	animal, plants
Oleic Acid, omega-9	18	1	animal, plants
Linoleic Acid, omega-6	18	2	animal, plants
Linolenic Acid, omega 3	18	3	animal, plants
Arachidonic Acid, omega-6	20	4	animal, plants
Eicospentenoic Acid, omega-3	20	5	mainly fish
Docosahexenoic Acid, omega-3	22	6	mainly fish

*From Marinetti, G.V. 1990, chapter 1, Table 1-1 page 8 with kind permission of Springer Science and Business Media. The designations omega-3, omega-6, and omega-9 refer to the number of the carbon atom from the most distal double bond to the methyl terminal end of the fatty acid chain. The double bonds in natural fatty acids in humans have the cis configuration. Some researchers use the Greek symbol ω to designate omega in place of the letter n. Today, the small letter n is replacing the word omega. However, the labeling of many foods and fish oils for the public prefers to use the word omega.

The importance of the dietary trans fatty acids and the omega-3 (n-3) versus the omega-6 (n-6) fatty acids in health, heart disease and cancer are discussed in Chapters 2 and 3. I shall use the designation n-3, n-6, and n-9 in the chapters that follow.

Hydrogenation of vegetable oils to produce margarines converts some of the natural cis double bonds to the unnatural trans double bond. The cis double bond allows the fatty acid to have a more linear structure whereas the trans double bond makes the fatty acid have a puckered structure. The fatty acids with trans double bonds are incorporated into cell membranes and may alter the structure and function of the membrane lipid bilayer in an unfavorable manner. This may in part explain how dietary trans fatty acids increase blood cholesterol levels and increase the risk of heart disease in humans.

Today most manufacturers have eliminated or have reduced the amount of trans fats in margarines, baked goods, cereals, and other foods. This wise move will protect many humans from the risk of heart disease.

Eicosapentenoic acid (EPA) and docosahexenoic acid (DHA) are commonly referred to as omega-3 (or n-3) fatty acids. These two fatty acids are found primarily in fish oils and are receiving much attention today as important dietary supplements. Fish obtain these two fatty acids from eating plankton in the oceans or lakes.

Fatty acids that have no double bonds are called saturated fatty acids. Fatty acids with one double bond are called monounsaturated fatty acids; those with two or more double bonds are called polyunsaturated fatty acids (PUFAs).

Knowledge of how the body digests and absorbs dietary lipids, carbohydrates and proteins is essential to have a better understanding of metabolism. The main dietary lipids are triglycerides (fats) that are found in foods like butter, cheese, margarines, ice cream, pie crust, peanut butter, many cookies and muffins, fatty steaks, egg yolk, and salad dressings containing vegetable oils like corn oil, olive oil, peanut oil, safflower oil, canola oil and other vegetable oils. Triglycerides contain both saturated and unsaturated fatty acids. Chapter 1 discusses how foods are digested, obesity and the metabolic syndrome. The metabolic syndrome is a risk factor for type-2 diabetes and heart disease and is an important health topic today in nutrition.

Part 2

Digestion of Foods, Diets and Drug Treatments for Heart Disease, and the History of Atherosclerosis

Chapter 1

Digestion of Foods, Obesity and the Metabolic Syndrome

Digestion of Lipids

Starting this chapter on the digestion of foods will provide background information of how the foods are broken down and then absorbed into the blood. The absorbed foods are then either oxidized to provide energy and heat for the body or are used to make new lipids, proteins, and carbohydrates. Excess fat is stored in fat cell and the excess carbohydrate is stored as glycogen in the liver. Fat cells have a great capacity to store fat. In contrast, the liver has a limited capacity to store carbohydrate. The process of digestion and absorption of foods requires special enzymes and is regulated by several hormones such as insulin, glucagon, and epinephrine (adrenalin).

The digestion of dietary fats (mainly triglycerides) begins in the mouth by the action of an enzyme called lingual lipase. The stomach contains an acid lipase that also hydrolyzes triglycerides. These acid lipases hydrolyze triglycerides to diglycerides and fatty acid. The lingual and gastric lipases are more important in infants because they consume large quantities of milk in which the triglycerides are highly emulsified. Salivary and gastric lipases are believed to account for about 10–20 percent hydrolysis of triglycerides in adults and about 40–50 percent in infants.

The most important lipase that digests fats is pancreatic lipase. Fat absorption is very efficient. Most fat is digested in the proximal (upper) region of the small intestine but with heavy intake of fat the absorption may extend to the distal (lower) region of the small intestines. The saturated fats are digested and absorbed less well than the unsaturated fats. The digestion of fats is regulated by several hormones.

Fatty acid salts are soaps and help emulsify the fats in the intestines. The fatty acids also stimulate the gallbladder to contract allowing bile to flow into the small intestine. Bile is released into the intestines about 5–10 times per day. Peristalsis promotes the movement of the digested foods through the intestines. The digested lipids are absorbed by lymphatic ducts that allow the digestion products to get into the blood stream where they enter the liver and are converted to lipoproteins called chylomicrons. Pancreatic lipase requires colipase for full activity. Colipase is a small protein that is required for the binding of pancreatic lipase to emulsified triglyceride particles. Other lipases hydrolyze dietary phospholipids, glycolipids, and cholesterol esters.

Dietary cholesterol esters are hydrolyzed in the small intestine by pancreatic cholesterol esterase to produce free cholesterol and fatty acid. Bile salts are also required for emulsification of the water-insoluble cholesterol and cholesterol esters.

Chylomicrons give the blood a milky appearance which can last for several hours after eating a high fat diet. Since the most abundant dietary lipids are triglycerides, the major lipid digestion products are monoglycerides and free fatty acids as shown in the figure below in Figure 1.1.

Figure 1.1 Hydrolysis of triglycerides by pancreatic lipase

Triglycerides ——————> Monoglycerides + 2 Fatty Acids

Monoglycerides ——————> Glycerol + Fatty Acids

The products of lipid digestion are absorbed in the small intestines. Within the intestinal mucosal cells, the fatty acids and monoglycerides are converted back to triglycerides and phospholipids that have different arrangement of the fatty acids than those from the diet. The absorbed lipids along with phospholipids and cholesterol are packaged with specific proteins to form lipoproteins.

Milk triglycerides have a relatively high content of fatty acids of shorter chain length. In contrast, vegetable and animal triglycerides contain very little or no shorter chain fatty acids. The shorter chain fatty acids are absorbed directly into the blood and are not converted to chylomicrons. This is important for persons who have high levels of triglycerides and need to eat fewer fats. The lipid digestion products enter the blood where they are analyzed to be sure the levels are in the normal range. The lipid content of human plasma is shown in the table below in Table 1.1.

Table 1.1 Lipid content of human plasma*

Lipid Type	Mean (mg/dl)	Range (mg/dl)
Total lipid	570	360–820
Triglycerides	142	80–180
Total Phospholipid	215	123–390
Phosphatidylcholine	175	50–200
Phosphatidylethanolamine	90	50–130
Sphingomyelin	25	15–35
Total cholesterol	200	107–320
Free Cholesterol	55	26–106
Free Fatty Acids	12	6–16

*From Murray et al 1988 with permission and from Marinetti, G.V. 1990 Chapter 1, Table 1.2, page 24 with permission of Springer Science and Business Media. The mean values and range for the phospholipids were calculated by G. Marinetti. Plasma is the super-natant fluid obtained by centrifuging whole blood.

The table shows that human plasma has a variety of lipids. The lipids that are most often analyzed are total cholesterol and triglycerides. The lipid values are influenced by diet, hormones, age, sex, exercise, and other factors including drinking alcohol. Lipid analysis of plasma should be done after an overnight fast. This procedure is especially important for analysis of plasma triglycerides. After a very high fat meal, the triglyceride level of plasma can rise dramatically for a relatively short time period, reaching levels over 1000 mg/dl or more. Within six to eight hours the normal range of 50 to 150 mg/dl it reached.

Table 1.2 below shows the various lipases that occur in humans and animals.

Table 1.2 Lipases of human and animal origin*		
Lipase	**Origin**	**Function**
Gastric lipase	**Stomach**	**Degrades triglycerides**
Pancreatic lipase	**Pancreas**	**Degrades triglycerides**
Lipoprotein lipase	**Non-liver tissues**	**Degrades triglycerides in chylomicrons and VLDL**
Hormone sensitive lipase	**Adipocytes**	**Degrades triglycerides**
Acid lipase	**Many cells**	**Degrades lipids taken up by lysosomes**
Hepatic lipase	**Liver**	**Degrades triglycerides in lipoprotein remnants**
Salivary lipase	**Mouth**	**Degrades triglycerides**

*From Patton and Hofmann, 1986 and from Marinetti, G.V. 1990 Table 1.2 Chapter 1, page 25 with kind permission and Springer Science and Business Media.

It is evident that lipases occur in different organs of the body and are not restricted to digestion of foods in the intestines. For examples acid lipases and hepatic lipase remove excess lipids in cells. Excess lipids in cells can damage the cells and cause diseases.

The fatty acids from the diet serve as a fuel for most cells of the body for energy production. The excess fatty acids are esterified to triglycerides and stored as fat droplets in adipose tissue (fat cells) or are esterified to phospholipids. Insulin stimulates the process of fat synthesis and storage. The hormone epinephrine stimulates the breakdown of stored fats.

During starvation or stress an adipose tissue lipase is activated by several hormones, notably epinephrine. Lipases hydrolyze the stored triglycerides and produce fatty acids that enter the blood. Insulin inhibits the fat cell lipase but stimulates fatty acid synthesis in adipose tissue and liver. Insulin also stimulates the entry and exit of glucose into fat cells.

Unlike triglycerides and phospholipids that have fatty acids that can be oxidized, cholesterol cannot be oxidized by the body. Cholesterol functions as an important component of cell membranes, as a precursor for adrenal steroid hormones, as a precursor for vitamin D in the skin, and as a substrate for the synthesis of bile acids in the liver.

Malabsorption of Digested Lipids

Malabsorption of digested lipids involves either defects in the breakdown of dietary lipids or impaired absorption of the digested lipids. These defects include impaired hydrolysis, impaired emulsification and over production of acid by the stomach. Impaired hydrolysis may be due to a deficiency of pancreatic lipase or colipase.

A deficiency of bile acids causes impaired emulsification of the dietary triglycerides. High acidity in the small intestine is caused by a deficiency of bicarbonate production by the pancreas. Sodium bicarbonate is alkaline and is needed to neutralize the excess acid produced by the stomach. Excess acid makes the intestine too acidic and inhibits pancreatic lipase. Some causes of impaired hydrolysis of dietary triglycerides are shown below in Table 1.3.

Table 1.3 Causes of impaired digestion of dietary triglycerides*	
Abnormality	**Occurs in**
Pancreatic lipase deficiency	**Pancreatitis and cystic fibrosis**
Excess stomach acid	**Stomach cancer (Gastrinoma)**
Decreased secretion of bicarbonate by the pancreas	**Chronic pancreatitis**
Decreased colipase secretion	**Colipse deficiency**

*From Patton and Hofmann, 1986 reproduced with permission and from Marinetti, G.V. 1990 Chapter 1, Table 1.4 page 28 with kind permission of Springer Science and Business Media.

When bile is deficient as a result of severe liver dysfunction, fat digestion and absorption are markedly impeded and fat accumulates in the feces. This condition is called steatorrhea. The accumulated fats consist of fatty acid salts and undigested triglycerides. Malabsorption can lead to deficiencies of the fat-soluble vitamins A, D, E, and K. The consequences of pancreatic lipase and bile acid deficiency are shown below in Table 1.4.

Table 1.4 Consequences of pancreatic lipase and bile acid deficiency*	
Deficiency	**Consequences**
Pancreatic lipase or Bile acids	**Steatorrhea, loss of dietary fat, loss of fat soluble vitamins A, D, E, K, weight loss, diarrhea, and death**

*From Patton and Hofmann, 1986 reproduced with permission and from Marinetti, G.V. 1990 Chapter 1, Table 1.5, page 28 with kind permission of Springer Science and Business Media.

If the pancreas is damaged or inflamed (as in pancreatitis) or if the pancreatic duct is obstructed, pancreatic enzymes will not be made or will not be released, and a deficiency of pancreatic lipase occurs. The deficiency of pancreatic lipase or colipase gives rise to a fatty steatorrhea consisting mainly of undigested triglycerides. This condition also can lead to severe weight loss and the loss of the vitamins A, D, E, and K.

Bacteria normally found in the colon hydrolyze some of the undigested triglycerides and cause a fatty acid diarrhea. Patients with this problem are treated with a dried pancreas product called Pancreatin, which contains lipases, proteases, and amylase. Care must be used to give the proper dose depending on the amount and type of food in the diet at any one time. Large amounts of acidic vitamin C and chondroitin sulfate can decrease the effect of Pancreatin. Also taking excess Metamucil with the Pancreatin can bind some of the enzymes and bile acids and decreases the effectiveness of these enzymes.

Damaged or inflamed mucosal cells (that can occur in celiac disease in children and in sprue in adults) interfere with absorption of the products of lipid digestion and give rise to steatorrhea and lead to vitamin deficiency. In these cases, the major lipid in the feces consists of fatty acid salts. Sprue is caused by a severe allergy to the protein gluten found in many wheat products.

Decreased bile acid secretion may occur with liver disease. A deficiency of bile acids leads to impaired emulsification of the dietary fat. The undigested fats cause impaired fat absorption, loss of weight, and diarrhea. Unabsorbed fats alone do not cause diarrhea. However, bacteria produce hydroxylated fatty acids that have a direct stimulatory effect on the colon that leads to diarrhea.

Bile salt deficiency, lipase deficiency, and decreased or defective mucosa (lining of the intestine) cause fat malabsorption and diarrhea. Severe diarrhea causes dehydration and acidosis, which can be life threatening, especially to infants and children. The acidosis (a severe acidity of the blood) results from a loss of sodium and potassium from the small intestine. When the acidity of the blood pH (a scale used to identify acidity or alkalinity) falls below 7.0, coma and death can result. The normal pH of the blood is 7.35–7.45.

Digestion of Carbohydrates: the Glycemic Index.

Digestion of dietary carbohydrates from starch, potato, rice, and pasta is carried out primarily in the small intestine by the enzyme pancreatic amylase. A salivary amylase breaks down some starches to smaller fragments. These carbohydrates are digested rapidly and converted to the sugar call glucose. The glucose is absorbed readily into the blood by a process called active transport. The blood sugar rises and signals the pancreas to make insulin that gets to the liver and stimulates the conversion of glucose to a polymer called glycogen. This lowers the blood glucose level back to normal which is between 70–110 mg/dl.

However, carbohydrates in vegetables and fruits are digested more slowly and do not raise the blood sugar level as much. **The glycemic index of carbohydrates is based on how high the level of blood glucose and blood insulin gets when a given amount of the carbohydrate is ingested. Table sugar has a high glycemic index.**

Table sugar (sucrose) is hydrolyzed by the enzyme sucrase, milk sugar lactose is hydrolyzed by lactase, and malt sugar is hydrolyzed by maltase. These enzymes occur in the small intestines. Some persons lack the enzyme lactase and suffer from abdominal pain and bloating that comes from the overproduction of gas that is produced by bacterial fermentation in the colon (the large intestine). These persons now can drink lactase-treated milk called Lactaid.

Persons who consume a large amount of potato, refined rice, or refined pasta cause the blood sugar level to rise above normal. This in turn causes the pancreas to produce more than the normal amount of insulin that rapidly converts the glucose to glycogen. If this process occurs too rapidly, the blood glucose level will fall rapidly and a person can develop a low level of blood glucose (hypoglycemia) and feel faint.

Continued long term eating of excess refined carbohydrates such as potato, rice, and pasta may overstress the pancreas to produce too much insulin and wear out the pancreas and cause type-2 diabetes. The stress on the pancreas may lead to insulin resistance that is manifested by the decreased ability of insulin to regulate the blood sugar level. This condition causes a persistent elevation of blood glucose which over time allows the glucose to attach to some proteins that alter the normal function of these proteins. If this occurs on blood vessels it damages the blood vessels and leads to poor circulation or leaky vessels and if it occurs in the retina it can cause the wet type of macular degeneration that can lead to blindness.

Overeating refined carbohydrates causes overweight and eventually causes obesity. Today obesity among children and adults is a major health problem because it predisposes these individuals to diabetes and heart disease.

Insulin is necessary not only to form glycogen in the liver but also to form and store triglycerides in fat cells. Long term feeding of bad carbohydrates coupled with high levels of blood insulin leads to excess fat in fat cells and to an increase in the number of fat cells that cause overweight and obesity. Hormones called leptin and ghrelin regulate fat metabolism and are involved in obesity.

Digestion of Proteins

Digestion of proteins occurs by the enzyme pepsin in the stomach, by the pancreatic enzymes trypsin and chymotrypsin, and by dipeptidases in the small intestine that ultimately produce amino acids. The amino acids are absorbed into the blood. The absorbed amino acids are used by the organs of the body for the synthesis of new proteins. The end products of protein degradation in the body are urea and ammonia.

The next section considers what may happen when persons eat too much food and gain weight and the role of the protein factors called leptin and ghrelin in this process.

Obesity: The Role of Leptin and Ghrelin

Leptin is a protein with hormone activity that regulates metabolism of body fat. The treatment of obese mice, which are genetically deficient in leptin, with gene therapy results in reduction in both food intake and body weight. Leptin may play a role in regulating insulin levels in the blood. Treatment of the obese mice with leptin gene therapy led to the normalization of blood insulin levels and glucose tolerance. These studies suggest that leptin may be used for the control of body weight and for the management of type 2 diabetes.

The hormone ghrelin also regulates food intake. The principal site of ghrelin synthesis is the stomach. Ghrelin is believed to regulate food intake by acting on the pituitary growth hormone. Ghrelin may be an endocrine link between stomach, hypothalamus and pituitary gland and thus plays a role in the regulation of energy balance and weight control.

Among U.S. adults aged 20–40 years, the prevalence of overweight (BMI 25–30) has increased in 1980 from by 33–35 percent in the U.S. population. In the same population, obesity (defined as BMI greater than or equal to 30) has nearly doubled from approximately 15 percent in 1980 to an estimated 33 percent by 2005. This has led to an increase in type 2 diabetes during this time interval. And it appears to be increasing up to the present time. Overweight refers to increased body weight in relation to height, when compared to some standard of acceptable weight Acceptable weights relative to height for men and women are listed in the table below in Table 1.5.

	Men	Women
Height (feet—inches)	**Acceptable range (lbs)**	**Acceptable range (lbs)**
4' 9"		99–128
4' 10"		100–131
4' 11"		101–134
5' 0"		103–137
5' 1"	123–145	105–140
5' 2"	125–148	108–143
5' 3"	127–151	111–148
5' 4"	129–155	114–152
5' 5"	131–159	117–156
5' 6"	133–163	120–16-
5' 7"	135–167	123–164
5' 8"	137–171	126–167
5' 9"	139–175	129–170
5' 10"	141–179	132–173
5' 11"	144–183	135–176
6' 0"	147–187	
6' 1"	150–192	
6' 2"	153–197	
6' 3"	157–202	

Table 1.5 Acceptable weights for men and women by height*

*Weights are without clothes and heights are without shoes. Taken from the Metropolitan Life Insurance Co., 1983.(Source of basic data 1979 Build Study of Actuaries and Association of Life Insurance Medical Directors of America 1980)/

Overweight may or may not be due to increases in body fat. It may also be due to an increase in lean muscle. For example, professional athletes may be very lean and muscular, with very little body fat, yet they may weigh more than others of the same height. While they may qualify as "overweight" due to their large muscle mass, they are not obese.

Obesity, the Metabolic Syndrome and Type 2 Diabetes

Obesity is the accumulation of excess fat (triglycerides) and excess number of fat cells in adipose tissue of the body that leads to excess weight accumulation. Insulin plays a role in obesity by regulating how fats are stored, mobilized, and oxidized by cells. Obesity and diabetes predispose persons to atherosclerosis, heart disease and stroke.

Determinants of the Metabolic Syndrome

The risk for CAD can be reduced beyond lowering the blood LDL cholesterol level by modification of other risk factors. One major target is the metabolic syndrome, which represents a constellation of lipid and non-lipid risk factors of metabolic origin. This syndrome is closely linked to a general metabolic disorder called insulin resistance in which the normal actions of insulin are impaired. Persons with antibodies to insulin or to the insulin receptors or to faulty insulin receptors are in this category.

Excess body fat, in particular (abdominal fat) and physical inactivity promote the development of insulin resistance. The determinants that are used in the diagnosis of the metabolic syndrome are shown in Table 1.6.

Table 1.6 Determinants of the metabolic syndrome	
Risk Factor	**Defining Level**
Abdominal obesity Men Women	**Waist Circumference** >102 cm (40 in) > 88 cm (35 in)
Triglyceride level mg/dl	> 150
HDL cholesterol mg/dl Men Women	< 40 < 50
Blood Pressure, mm Hg	> 130 systolic; > 85 diastolic,
Fasting Glucose mg/dl	> 110

Persons with the metabolic syndrome have excess abdominal fat, high levels of blood triglycerides, low levels of good HDL cholesterol, high blood pressure, and elevated fasting glucose levels above 110 mg/dl. These persons do not exercise enough; they eat excess refined carbohydrates, become resistant to insulin, and may in later life get type-2 diabetes.

Obesity and Body Mass Index (BMI)

Obesity is defined as an excessively high amount of body fat or adipose tissue in relation to lean body mass. The amount of body fat includes both the distribution of fat throughout the body and the size of the adipose tissue. Body fat distribution can be estimated by skin fold measures, waist-to-hip circumference ratios, or techniques such as ultrasound, computed tomography, or magnetic resonance imaging.

BMI is the ratio of weight-to-height. It uses a mathematical formula in which a person's body weight in kilograms is divided by the square of his or her height in meters (wt/ht^2). The BMI is more highly correlated with body fat than with height and weight

Individuals with a BMI of 25 to 29.9 are considered overweight, while individuals with a BMI of 30 or more are considered obese. According to the *NIH Clinical Guidelines on the Identification, Evaluation and the Treatment of Overweight and Obesity in Adults* (aged 18 years or older) persons who have a BMI of 25 or more are considered at risk for premature death and disability. These health risks increase even more as the severity of an individual's obesity increases.

Overweight and Obesity in Children and Adolescents

The percentage of children and adolescents who are defined as overweight has more than doubled since the early 1970s. About 13 percent of children and adolescents are now seriously overweight. In spite of the public health impact of obesity and overweight, these conditions have not been a major public health priority in the past. Halting and reversing the upward trend of the obesity epidemic will require effective collaboration among government, voluntary, and private sectors, as well as a commitment to action by individuals and communities across the nation.

Measurement of Waist Circumference

With a tape measure, comfortably measure the distance around the smallest area below the rib cage and the area above the umbilicus (belly button).

Measurement of Hip Circumference

With a tape measure, comfortably measure the distance around the largest extension of the buttocks. Waist circumference is a common measure used to assess abdominal fat content. The presence of excess body fat in the abdomen, when out of proportion to total body fat, is considered an independent predictor of risk factors and ailments associated with obesity.

Undesirable waist circumferences differ for men and women. Men are at risk who have a waist measurement greater than 40 inches (102 cm) Women are at risk who have a waist measurement greater than 35 inches (88 cm) If a person has short stature (under five feet in height) or has a BMI of 35 or above, waist circumference standards used for the general population may not apply.

Waist-to-hip ratio (WHR) is the ratio of a person's waist circumference to hip circumference, mathematically calculated as the waist circumference divided by the hip circumference. For most people carrying extra weight around their middle increases health risks more than carrying extra weight around their hips or thighs. (Overall obesity is still more risky than body fat storage locations or waist-to-hip ratio.) For both men and women, a waist-to-hip ratio of 1.0 or higher is considered "at risk" or in the danger zone for undesirable health consequences, such as heart disease and diabetes. For men, a ratio of .90 or less is considered safe. For women, a ratio of .80 or less is considered safe. The next chapter 2 discusses diets for lowering the levels of blood cholesterol and triglycerides to decrease the risk of getting heart disease.

See chapter 5 for fatty acid metabolism and chapter 9 for information on how excess carbohydrates are converted to fats and cause obesity.

Chapter 2

Dietary Therapy for High Levels of Blood Lipids

High levels of blood cholesterol, in particular LDL-cholesterol, are associated with premature atherosclerosis and heart disease. Therefore, it is important to know how drug therapy and dietary management can be used to lower blood cholesterol levels. The effect of dietary management is considered first, since for most people this approach to treatment of hyperlipidemia is tried before drug therapy.

The public in the US is informed by the *American Heart Association* and other agencies on the effect of nutrition on heart disease. Early recommendations by the *American Heart Association* on decreasing total fat intake to 30 percent or less without considering the type of fat (saturated versus polyunsaturated) made matters worse since this led many persons to eat more carbohydrate and gain weight.

Fortunately this has been rectified with the newer knowledge on the benefit of polyunsaturated n-3 fat and the danger of eating too much refined carbohydrates found in white rice, most pastas, and potatoes. This effort has led to very significant changes in the eating habits of Americans who are now are consuming less beef, pork, hamburgers, fried potatoes, and hotdogs and eating more chicken, turkey, and fish.

Restriction of dietary intake of saturated fatty acids and trans fatty acids is important in reducing plasma cholesterol levels. Saturated fatty acids occur in high amounts in dairy products, bacon fat, and lard, coconut oil, and palm oil. Trans fatty acids are found in many hydrogenated fats such as margarines and in baked goods.

The degree of reduction of LDL-cholesterol levels that can be achieved by dietary therapy depends on a person's eating habits before the diet is started and on the inherent responsiveness of the person based on the person's genetic makeup. In general, people with high cholesterol levels show a greater absolute reduction in total and LDL-cholesterol levels than do those with relatively low or normal cholesterol levels.

Diets Proposed To Prevent Heart Disease and Obesity

More than 44 million people are clinically obese compared with 30 million a decade ago. This puts these persons at risk for heart disease, stroke, and diabetes. A severe national health crisis is pending in the US unless steps are taken now to lower the growing number of obese children and adults. This can be done by combined therapy using diets, exercise, and drugs. Diet and exercise therapy should be tried first and drugs should be used only if diet and exercise therapies are not successful.

In the final analysis the laws of thermodynamics prevail. Thermodynamics is the study of the dynamics of heat and energy transfer. It is a very well studied field of physics which has led to the development of engines that are used in our everyday lives but also applies to living systems.

To maintain a steady weight, the amount of food calories consumed in the diet must equal the amount of calories burned by or lost by the body. Weight gain occurs when the amount of food calories consumed in the diet exceeds the amount of calories burned or lost by the body. To lose weight the amount of food calories consumed in the diet must be less than the amount of calories lost by the body. Overeating and lack of exercise cause weight gain. Other factors such as illness, cancer, vitamin deficiency, mineral deficiency, and genetic abnormalities will influence weight gain or loss.

Shown below are some diets in the US for treating obesity and high levels of blood cholesterol and triglycerides. Not all these diets are effective or recommended. The Dr. Willett and the Dr. Ornish diets are the best ones based on sound science.

The material in Table 2.1 and Table 2.2 shown below and information on the studies of Dr. Willet et al. have been taken and modified from the article by *Lemley, B.," What Does Science Say You Should Eat?, Discover Magazine, Feb. 2004, pp. 43–49.* Mr. B. Lemley has kindly given permission to use this material.

Table 2.1 Diets for treating obesity and high levels of blood lipids*
Dr. Atkins diet—high in meats and fats, low in carbohydrates
Dr. Ornish diet—a balanced diet high in vegetables and fiber
Grapefruit, rice, protein diet
Scarsdale diet—14 day diet, eat until satisfied, no sugar, cream, honey, substitute fish and poultry for red meats, follow a 14 day schedule
Beverly Hills diet—high in nuts, fruits, pineapple juice, alternate carbohydrate with protein
Best Chance diet low cholesterol, watch calories and avoid stress
Eat Smart diet—7 days, eat more meals but with smaller portions of food
Miracle diet 48 hours liquid "Miracle juice" diet that contains fruits, vitamins, oils, and antioxidants
The new Dr. Willett diet is a balanced common sense diet with good carbohydrates and good protein, plenty of nuts and vegetables, fish and poultry, less red meat, and less white carbohydrates.

*From Lemley, B. 2004 with kind permission.

The meat intensive diet of Dr. Robert Atkins differs greatly from the vegetarian diet of Dr. Dean Ornish. Another diet called the South Beach Diet is not shown in Table 2.1. The South Beach Diet consists of two phases and stresses good carbohydrates, avoids saturated fats, and recommends fish that contains the omega-3 fatty acids and also recommends olive oil.

Some Americans are tempted to follow Mark Twain's admonition to "eat what you like and let the food fight it out inside." (This statement is humorous but it is not a prudent policy for good nutrition).

I believe that diets should be based on sound science and should be simple and easy to follow. There is little need to weigh foods and carefully count calories. Eating should be enjoyable and just a common sense approach is needed. The Willett diet does this easily and effectively.

The Willett Diet: Based on Sound Science

The debate on what is the best nutrition continues but nutrition researchers have begun to form a consensus on a diet based on sound science. This diet has been proposed by Dr. Walter Willett, chairman of the department of nutrition at the *Harvard School of Public Health*. The Willett healthy eating plan has seven tiers indicated below in Table 2.2.

Table 2.2 Dr. Willett's diet*
Top tier no. 7 Use sparingly red meat, butter, white rice, white bread, potatoes, pasta, and sweets
Tier no. 6 Diary or calcium supplements 1 to 2 times a day
Tier no. 5 Fish, poultry, and eggs 0 to2 times a day
Tier no. 4 Nuts and legumes (beans) 1 to 3 times a day
Tier no. 3 Vegetables in abundance, fruits 2 to 3 times a day
Tier no. 2 Whole-grain foods and plant oils at most meals
Base Tier no. 1 Daily exercise and weight control

*From Lemley, B. 2004 with kind permission.

The Willett diet is depicted in a pyramid called the healthy eating pyramid, which has a common sense approach to diet. The base of the pyramid emphasizes daily exercise and weight control. **The Willett diet replaces the high carbohydrate, low fat diet with a good protein, good carbohydrate, and good fat diet. The Willett diet also allows for sparingly using refined rice, white bread, potatoes, pasta, and sweets that add to the enjoyment of eating.**

Good carbohydrates are those high in fiber and wheat that have a low glycemic index. Good fats are the n-3 fatty acids from fish oil and canola oil. Olive oil is also a good fat since it contains oleic acid. The benefits of oleic acid are discussed later in this chapter.

I question why in tier 5 Willett says 0–2 times a day for fish, poultry, and eggs. I would change this to the following: fish 3–4 times a week, poultry 2–3 times a week and no more than four whole eggs a week.

Prudent diets like the Willett diet have kept my weight normal and has kept my blood lipids normal (with the help of the drug Lipitor) for many years. I also suggest that eating smaller portions of food several times a day is preferred to eating a very large meal once a day. Also I advise avoid eating just before going to bed at night and eat the larger meal at noon if possible. This allows more time to burn off some of the food before going to bed.

The Willett diet resembles the Mediterranean that has been shown in several studies to reduce the risk of heart disease. The Mediterranean diet is specific to a certain climate and culture that focuses on healthy ingredients rather than on specific dishes.

The Willett diet is based on the largest long-term dietary survey ever undertaken. The 121,700 participant Nurses' Health Study began in 1976 by Harvard professor Frank Speizer and with dietary assessments supervised by Dr. Willett since 1980. Willett crafted it so that he and others could extract specific recommendations about food intake. Participants gave blood and toenail samples so that information was obtained on the absorption of trace elements and other nutrients. This study included both sexes and two generations of subjects. **Dr. Willett's group launched the Health Professionals Follow-UP Study, which included 52,000 men and the Nurses Health study II a survey of 116,000 younger women.**

The earlier low fat diets in the US actually made people eat more bad carbohydrates and gain weight. Excess carbohydrate in the diet is converted to fat, which is stored in fat tissue. Excess carbohydrate also causes insulin levels in the blood to increase that promotes the storage of fat, increases body weight.

Soft drinks containing high levels of sugar are to be restricted or avoided by children and adults. The sugars in soft drinks have a high glycemic index. Children and adults who drink soft drinks daily put a stress on the pancreas to produce insulin and also tend to gain weight. Soft drinks containing sugar substitutes are available but the long term (30 to 40 years) effects of sugar substitutes remain to be determined by large controlled clinical studies.

Overeating refined starches found in white four, pasta, potato, and consuming excess table sugar leads to an increase in amylase secretion by the pancreas. Amylase is an important digestive enzyme that converts complex dietary carbohydrate to glucose. Elevated levels of amylase cause blood glucose levels to increase that then stimulate the pancreas to produce insulin. After many years of insulin overload, the cells of the body may become resistant to insulin.

Blood glucose levels remain elevated over a long time period since the blunting of insulin's normal function prevents the excess glucose from being stored as glycogen and favors it being converted to fat. **Over time the stress on the pancreas may lead to type 2-diabetes. Obesity also can give rise to the metabolic syndrome that predisposes persons to type-2 diabetes.** See chapter 1 for more information on the metabolic syndrome.

The Willett diet advises eating vegetables in abundance, consuming alcohol in moderation, and taking a daily multivitamin to cover nutritional gaps. His diet also recommends eating fish as a source of protein and eating the heart protective n-3 fatty acids (EPA and DHA). Those who worry about mercury contamination in fish may get some relief from a recent study at the University of Rochester Medical School.

This study tracked pregnant women who ate an average of 12 fish meals a week about 10 times the quantity of fish eaten by the average American. This study found no evidence that low levels of mercury in seafood are harmful. Moreover the women's children suffered no adverse cognitive, behavioral or neurological effects. The question still remains however, were these sufficiently long term studies. Moreover, the types of fish (i.e. salt water versus fresh water fish) consumed and where and how they were obtained are important.

Dr. Willett also recommends the importance of exercise and states that the best choice for many, especially the elderly and persons suffering from arthritis, is walking exercise. The Nurse's study revealed a strong link between walking and protection against heart disease. **Women who walked an average of three hours a week (about 30 minutes a day) were 35 percent less likely to have a heart attack over an eight year period compared to those women who walked less.** The benefits of walking daily are covered in a later section of this chapter.

Other foods to be used sparingly by the Willett diet are hydrogenated fats and trans fats found in shortening, margarines, deep fried foods, and packaged baked goods including cereals, crackers, potato chips, and cookies. Fortunately today many margarines and food products contain no trans fatty acids. **Trans fatty acids are more injurious than saturated fatty acids as a risk factor for heart disease.**

Willett counsels that dairy products like whole milk (and cheese) that supply a lot of calories from saturated fat are not the best way to get dietary calcium. He recommends a daily intake of 1200 mg of calcium for adults over 50. Eating calcium rich vegetables like leafy greens is recommended.

The Diets and Supplements that My Wife and I Use

Most medical doctors are hesitant to recommend dietary supplements for their patients. They are trained to accept only drugs that have been tested in good controlled clinical studies and approved by the FDA. Also doctors swear an oath to do no harm to their patients. This makes them proceed with great caution especially if they may be sued by their patients. I agree with this but also believe that I can take chances on taking dietary supplements if there is a sound scientific reason to do so. Also I do not have to fear being sued.

I do take some of these supplements if there is some sound biochemical basis to do so. I also inform my doctor before taking these supplements and give him my reasons based on my knowledge of biochemistry. My doctor and I agree that taking reasonable doses of the supplements is acceptable and they may offer some benefit and are likely to do no harm.

My wife and I use olive oil and canola oil mixtures for salads and cooking poultry. I try to eat fish (salmon and cod) twice a week. We also take fish oil capsules containing 1200 mg of the omega-3 fatty acids EPA and DHA three to four times a week. This provides a balance of the monounsaturated fatty acids and polyunsaturated fatty acids especially the n-3 polyunsaturated fish fatty acids. We use the high wheat, high fiber, low carbohydrate pasta and wheat breads (that have a low glycemic index) in place of white pasta and white breads. Our daily diet consists of a balance of vegetables, fruits, nuts (walnuts), and proteins from fish, turkey, and chicken.

We also take the following supplements daily: aspirin (325 mg for me and 81 mg for my wife), folic acid (400 micrograms), natural vitamin E (400 Internat. units). We take a one a day multi-vitamins pill (containing all the vitamins and essential minerals) three times a week.

In addition, because I had heart surgery for coronary artery disease I take one pill each of L-carnitine (250 mg), CoQ-10 (30 mg), and alpha-Lipoic acid (30 mg) every other day. My reason for taking these supplements is based on my knowledge of biochemistry and on the research of biochemist Dr. Ames. I emphasize that long term clinical studies have not yet been done to prove their health value. Studies by Dr. Ames on rats shows that carnitine and lipoic acid protect rats from oxidative damage and increase their life span. It is hoped that similar results will be found in humans.

My wife and I have a family history of heart disease and unknowingly had high levels of blood cholesterol and triglycerides for many years. To treat our high levels of blood lipids we take daily 20 mg of the statin drug Lipitor. This drug inhibits the key enzyme step in the synthesis of cholesterol and has controlled our blood lipids very well.

However, the inhibition of cholesterol synthesis also may inhibit the synthesis of isoprene compounds needed to make isoprenoids for the synthesis of CoQ-10. Thus long term use of Lipitor may lead to a deficiency of CoQ-10 that is needed to oxidized foods by the mitochondria. Furthermore carnitine is needed to allow fatty acids to enter the mitochondria so they can be oxidized. I point out that to my knowledge; no clinical studies have been done to prove the benefits of supplements such as L-carnitine, folic acid, and CoQ-10. However, studies on the health benefits of statins like Lipitor have been established by clinical studies on humans.

A deficiency of carnitine has been found in humans and it causes muscle weakness and allows triglycerides to accumulate in muscles. Since skeletal muscle and heart muscle prefer to oxidize fatty acids, a deficiency of carnitine and CoQ-10 may well lead to muscle weakness in both skeletal muscle and heart muscle. Such a deficiency eventually may damage the muscles and mitochondria of these organs. This is speculation on my part but is based on sound science.

The well known biochemist, Dr. Bruce Ames, professor of *Biochemistry and Molecular Biology at the University of California* in Berkeley and coworkers have done many studies with rats that show mitochondrial damage occurs with aging and that taking supplements such as L-acetyl-carnitine (or L-carnitine) and alpha-acid prevent premature aging by improving metabolic function and protecting against oxidative damage and mitochondrial decay in aging.

Alpha lipoic acid is a coenzyme of the mitochondrial enzyme pyruvate dehydrogenase which converts pyruvic acid to acetyl-CoA for oxidation by the mitochondria. This enzyme is highly regulated and controls how glucose and fatty acids are oxidized to produce energy. Lipoic acid deficiency may have harmful effects on mitochondrial function and may damage heart muscle.

The proper dose of each supplement has yet to be determined. One should use common sense for the time being. It is not necessary to follow the dose recommended by the manufactures of these supplements since I believe they are too high and expensive. Keep in mind that these supplements act like vitamins and like most vitamins (except for vitamin C) they are required in small amounts.

Thus there is uncertainty in the proper dosage to take, but taking small amounts should be safe and are unlikely to do harm. Some argue that by eating a healthy diet there is no need to take these supplements or vitamins. This may pertain to young persons who eat well, but with age most biochemical systems are believed to slow down, including the digestion and absorption of foods. Much more research is needed in this area of nutrition. The *National Institutes of Health* has now started research on herbs as supplements in order to remove the guessing on how effective they may or may not be.

The potential benefit of herbs is based on Chinese history and relies heavily on word of mouth experience from generation to generation. This type of evidence is not based on hard science and thus we await the studies from the

NIH. However, the thousands of years of experience from the Chinese with herbs cannot be dismissed out of hand.

Folic acid has been shown to protect humans from plaque formation in arteries resulting from high blood levels of blood homocystine that is an inflammatory compound on blood vessels. Folic acid helps degrade homocystine and is now recommended as a supplement for persons at risk for atherosclerosis and heart disease. One aspirin pill a day has been shown by the large study from Harvard University to offer protection from heart attacks.

I buy fish oil capsules in which the fish oil has been extracted from the muscles and not from the liver. The liver of fish tends to concentrate contaminants found in the sea. Call the company that sells the fish oil capsules to be certain how the fish oil is prepared.

Plant Sterols Lower the Level of Blood Lipids

Vegetables contain plant sterols called sitosterol and ergosterol. Some studies have shown that these plant sterols inhibit the absorption of cholesterol in the blood and may lower blood cholesterol levels. However, large controlled long term clinical studies in humans on the benefits of taking these sterols have not yet been done. Some non-prescription drugs containing plant sterols (such as Cholesterol Care) are available on the Internet and from Health Food stores. Also the statin drug Vytorin contains both a statin (Zocor) and ezetimbe (Zetia). Ezetimbe (Zetia) is a synthetic fluorinated sterol-like compound similar to the plant sterol beta-sitosterol. New drugs like the plant sterols may turn out to be effective at a lower cost in lowering blood lipids. However, will they lower blood lipid levels enough compared to the statin drugs? If future studies show they do lower blood lipids as well as the statins, this would be welcomed since the Statin drugs are expensive and are known to have bad side effects in some persons. However, to my knowledge long term controlled studies on humans using natural or synthetic sterols have not yet been done.

Vitamins: Functions and Deficiencies

All balanced diets should include the essential vitamins and minerals, essential amino acids, and essential fatty acids. In cases such as old age and illness is may be necessary to supplement the diets with vitamins. Vitamins are organic molecules, which the body cannot make. Therefore they must occur in the food that a person eats. The Table 2.3 below shows the main functions and defects caused by vitamin deficiencies.

Table 2.3 Dietary vitamins

Fat Soluble Vitamins	Function	Results of Deficiency
Vitamin A	Vision, cell differentiation Part of rhodopsin in the eye	Night Blindness
Vitamin D	Calcium and bone metabolism	Rickets, Osteomalacia
Vitamin E	Free radical scavenger Antioxidant	Lipid peroxidation, cell damage
Vitaminn K	Blood coagulation factors	Bleeding from pro- longed clotting time
Water soluble Vitamins	Function	Results of Deficiency
Thiamine	Enzyme decarboxylation, fat metabolism	Beriberi, heart failure
Riboflavin	Enzyme redox reactions for oxidation of foods	Weight loss, hyperkeratosis
Pantothenic acid	Fat metabolism, synthesis of coenzyme A for fat metabolism	Weight loss, fatigue Numbness
Niacin	Enzyme redox reactions in oxidation of foods	Pellagra, dermatitis, glossitis, blepharitis
Pyridoxine	Transamination reactions	Anemia
Biotin	Fatty acid metabolism	Dermatitis, alopecia (loss of hair)
Folic acid	Purine metabolism, syn- thesis of DNA and RNA	Megaloblastic anemia
Vitamin B-12	Homocysteine metabo- lism, DNA synthesis,	Perenicious Anemia, nerve degeneration
Vitamin C (ascorbic acid)	Collagen synthesis and maintain epithelial cells in skin, synthesis of dentine	Scurvy, bleeding gums, swelling of joints, weight loss

Vitamins act as coenzmes for the enzymes of the body and therefore play a vital role in the metabolism of foods. Deficiencies of any one vitamin, essential fatty acids, and essential amino acids will eventually lead to weight loss and death. High doses of vitamins A, D, and K can be very harmful.

Effects of Dietary Eggs and n-3 Fatty Acids on Blood Cholesterol Level

Dr. Willett defends eating eggs in moderation. However, I believe that eating eggs in excess (over 6 eggs a week) may raise blood cholesterol levels in susceptible persons. The diet and genetic makeup of the person will influence how many eggs a person can safely eat. Egg yolk contains good phospholipids that may help mobilize cholesterol in the blood. This effect (called by some the lipotropic effect) may offer some protection from the high cholesterol content in egg yolk, but I do not know of any good studies which support this idea.

Dietary manipulations to regulate serum cholesterol levels show great variability among individuals because of the unique genetic makeup and lifestyle of each person. The general conclusion, however, is that consumption of three or more eggs per day can increase serum LDL cholesterol levels in about 50 percent of persons with normal levels of blood cholesterol. The consumption of four eggs a week probably has little effect on the level of blood cholesterol for many persons.

The potential increase in blood cholesterol by eating too many eggs can be blunted by increasing the dietary n-3 fatty acids This can be done by ingesting polyunsaturated fatty acids found in fish (or fish oil capsules) and certain vegetable oils and avoiding the intake of foods rich in saturated fatty acids, such as butter, coconut oil, chocolate, pie crust, cream, and cakes and decreasing the trans fatty acids found in hydrogenated or partially hydrogenated foods like crackers, cereals and some margarines.

The most comprehensive study Willett and coworkers have assembled compared the health consequences of eating saturated fat versus unsaturated fat. A few researchers still question whether saturated fat is a risk factor for heart disease. One must take into account the number of patients studied, their ages, life styles, eating habits, exercise activity, and their ability to recall correct information on questionnaires used in the study. Diet studies on large number of humans are difficult and have many variable factors. The better studies on diets are those done in a hospital clinic under supervision. However, this type of study severely restricts the number of patients that can be used or who would participate and is much more expensive to carry out.

Dr. Willett points out that the amount of specific fats does make a difference. Women who ate more unsaturated fat had fewer heart problems. **Willett calculated that replacing five percent of saturated fat calories with unsaturated fat would cut the risk of heart attack and death by 40 percent.** The French Lyon Diet Heart Study of 1988 show a similar correlation.

The Benefit of Dietary Fiber

Dietary fiber also is important for lowering blood cholesterol. Fiber, which consists of complex carbohydrate polymers containing mucilage, pectins, lignin, and hemicelluloses, is found in plant foods such as grains, vegetables, legumes, fruits, (apples, pears, prunes), nuts, and seeds.

Fiber is divided into two types, soluble and insoluble. Insoluble fiber is coarse and chewy and is considered roughage. Soluble fiber is sticky like gums and gels. Fiber is not digested by humans, since humans lack the enzymes that degrade fiber. Insoluble fiber regulates bowel regularity by absorbing water and swelling. This softens the stool and stimulates the intestinal muscles to pass the stool through the intestine. Metamucil capsules are now available as a source of fiber. Eating vegetables high in fiber is preferable and more enjoyable than taking capsules.

Fibers are believed to lower blood cholesterol by binding bile acids and increasing their passage through the small intestines. Since most of the bile acids are absorbed in the small intestine, the less time food stays in the small intestine, the lower the amount of bile acids will be absorbed. The loss of bile acids then triggers the liver to convert more cholesterol to bile acids. This lowers the level of cholesterol in liver cell membranes that triggers the SREs (sterol regulatory elements) to make more LDL receptors on the liver cells, which makes the liver take up more cholesterol and converts it to bile acids. Thus the loss of bile acids from the intestines acts like a valve to drain cholesterol from the blood.

Soluble fiber appears to be more effective than insoluble fiber in lowering blood cholesterol. Soluble fiber found in corn bran, oat bran, carrots, and apples can reduce blood cholesterol. Usually, persons with higher cholesterol levels appear to get a greater reduction of cholesterol levels than do those with normal cholesterol levels. Reductions of blood cholesterol by up to twenty percent have been reported but usually this requires eating high amounts of foods rich in fiber.

To reduce blood cholesterol by fifteen to twenty percent, a substantial amount of fiber (three large bowls of oat bran per day) must be consumed. This type of diet is not practical. One cup of oat bran per day may lower blood cholesterol by approximately three percent. It is estimated that most Americans eat 10–15 g of total dietary fiber per day.

The *National Cancer Institute* and the *American Diabetes Association* encourage the eating of twenty to thirty grams of fiber per day. To get this latter amount of fiber, a person must consume three to five servings of whole-grain breads and cereals, three servings of vegetables, and two to three servings of fruit per day. A serving is considered to be two slices of whole grain bread, one medium piece of fruit, and one-half to two-thirds of a cup of vegetables daily.

Foods highest in fiber are black-eyed peas, kidney beans, bran, corn bran, oat bran, corn, peas, raw apples, prunes, barley, almonds, graham crackers, and corn bread. Recently products like Chitosol, Chitosan, and Metamucil are available to lower blood cholesterol. These plant-derived products bind bile acids and reduce cholesterol levels in the blood. From an economic point of view and eating pleasure, eating foods high in fiber is preferable to taking the more expensive supplements such as Chitosol, Chitosan, and Metamucil.

The Health Benefits of Eating Fish and Vegetable Oils

The n-3 and n-6 fatty acids are very important in health especially in protecting against heart disease and cancer. The n-3 fatty acids protect against these diseases whereas the n-6 fatty acids do not offer the same protection. The Table 2.4 below shows which foods have a high content of n-3 fatty acids or n-6 fatty acids.

Table 2.4 Dietary sources of n-3 and n-6 polyunsaturated fatty acids*	
Oils High in n-3 Fatty Acids	**Oils High in n-6 Fatty Acids**
Mainly fish and vegetable oils such as Salmon, Cod, Catfish, Mackerel , Haddak, Safflower, Corn, Canola, Cottonseed, Sunflower, Peanut	**Mainly animal fats such as beef, pork, and less so poultry**

*Modified from Goodnight et al. 1982 with permission and from Marinetti, G.V. 1990 Chapter 7, Table 7-5, page 140 with kind permission of Springer Science and Business Media.

Linolenic acid, eicosapentenoic acid (EPA), and docosahexenoic acid (DHA) are n-3 (omega-3) fatty acids. Arachidonic acid and linoleic acid are n-6 (omega-6) fatty acid. Fish oils contain the highest amount of EPA and DHA whereas vegetable oils have the highest content of linoleic acid and linolenic acid.

The n-3 fatty acid linolenic acid from vegetables has 18 carbon atoms. However the n-3 fatty acids from fish have 20 and 22 carbon atoms. These fatty acids may give rise to different eicosanoids which may have different biological functions in the body.

Vegetable oils have the highest content of the eighteen carbon n-3 fatty acids. Fish have the highest contents of n-3 eicosapentenoic acid (EPA) and n-3 docosahexenoic acid (DHA). Beef and pork have the highest content of n-6 fatty acid (arachidonic acid). On the other hand, Palm oil, coconut oil, beef, lard, and butter have the highest content of saturated fatty acids. Beef and pork have a high content of the n-6 arachidonic acid a precursor of the inflammatory prostaglandins.

Vegetable fats do not contain cholesterol but contain plant sterols (including sitosterol and ergosterol). Animal fats, especially beef, butter, liver, kidney, and sweetbreads (brain) contain high amounts of cholesterol. Animal fats usually contain less polyunsaturated fatty acids than do vegetable fats.

In addition to the value of n-3 fatty acids protecting against heart disease and cancer, the types of fatty acids are important since when taken in the diet they influence cholesterol levels, LDL and HDL levels in blood. **In general the n-3 fatty acids are more effective in lowering blood cholesterol levels, lowering the bad LDL cholesterol level, and increasing the good HDL cholesterol level than are the n-6 fatty acids. The trans fatty acids and the saturated fatty acids have opposite and bad effects on blood lipids.**

The fish n-3 fatty acids (EPA and DHA) protect not only from CAD and cancer but also protect against inflammation, thrombosis, and irregular heart beats (arrhythmias). The n-6 fatty acids are converted in part to the inflammatory prostaglandins. The n-3 fatty acids from fish inhibit the production of the n-6 fatty acids. Also fewer inflammatory prostaglandins are made from n-3 fatty acids than from n-6 fatty acids. These results clearly show the benefit of eating fish than eating beef and pork.

Vegetable fats do not contain cholesterol but have a variety of other plant sterols (including sitosterol and ergosterol). Animal fats, especially beef, butter, liver, kidney, and sweetbreads, contain relatively high amounts of cholesterol. Animal fats contain less polyunsaturated fatty acids than do vegetable fats.

The fatty acid content is important since the types of fatty acids taken in the diet determine whether these fatty acids lower, raise, or do not affect cholesterol levels and LDL and HDL levels in blood, how they influence the fluidity of cell membranes, and what type of prostaglandins they produce. The area of eicosanoids (prostaglandins, leukotrienes, and lipoxins) research is still in its infancy and I predict new studies will produce vital information on the important area of inflammation. The Table 2.5 below shows the types of fatty acids of plants ands animal fats.

Table 2.5 Types of fatty acids of plant and animal fats*
Vegetable oils high in polyunsaturated fatty acids: **Rapeseed, safflower, sunflower, corn, soybean, peanut, canola**
Vegetable oil high in monounsaturated fatty acid: **Olive oil**
Vegetable oils high in saturated fatty acids: **Palm. Coconut**
Animal fats high in saturated fatty acids: **Beef, lard, butter, pork**

From Marinetti, G.V. 1990 Chapter 7, Table 7-4, page 139 with kind permission of Springer Science and Business Media.

Cholesterol Content of Some Common Foods

The cholesterol content of some common foods is shown in the table below in Table 2.6.

Table 2.6 Cholesterol content of some common foods*	
Food	Cholesterol (mg)
Beef liver and kidney	440–700
Scallops	53
Oysters	45
Clams and lean fish	65
Shrimp	150
Chicken turkey white (light meat)t	80
Lobster	85
Beef lean	90
Chicken turkey dark meat	95
Egg yolk (one)	275

*From the US Department of Human Services, 1985. Based on 3.5 ounces of cooked meat; and from Marinetti, G.V. 1990 Chapter 7, Table 7.3, page 138 with kind permission of Springer Science and Business Media.

Beef liver and kidney have very high levels of cholesterol. Egg yolk also contains more cholesterol than other foods on a unit of weight basis. Surprisingly shrimp has high cholesterol content. This table is included because of the public interest in blood cholesterol levels as related to heart disease.

Effects of Dietary Oleic Acid (Olive Oil) on Blood Lipids

Substitution of monounsaturated and polyunsaturated fats (in proper amounts) for saturated fats in the diet has a lipid-lowering effect in most humans. The monounsaturated fatty acid, oleic acid (found in olive oil), has been shown to have the following beneficial effects: Oleic acid is the main fatty acid in olive oil that is used by people living in Mediterranean countries. **Listed below are some health benefits of oleic acid:**

1. decreases plasma LDL levels when substituted for saturated fatty acids.

2. decreases the risk of CAD.

3. does not promote carcinogenesis.

4. does not raise plasma triglyceride level.

5. does not lower plasma HDL level.

These findings were reported at the *Second Colloquium on Monounsaturates-Role of Monounsaturated Fatty Acids in Human Nutrition*, held on February 26, 1987, in Bethesda, Maryland.) The monounsaturated fatty acids cannot be converted to prostaglandins and leukotrienes, as can the n-3 or n-6 polyunsaturated fatty acids. Another potential benefit of monounsaturated fatty acids is their resistance to lipid peroxidation (Balasubramanian, et al, 1988, and Diplock, et al, 1988. Lipid peroxidation is a major cause of damage to cell membranes and also is believed to enhance carcinogenesis.

DHA (docosahexenoic acid), which occurs in fish, has been shown to increase the HDL/LDL ratio and protect humans from sudden death (Horrocks and Yeo 1999). They studied 20,000 male physicians over an 11 year period and found a 52 percent reduction in sudden death. The amount of n-3 fatty acids relative to n-6 fatty acids was critical. The beneficial effects were observed on lipid metabolism and on blood coagulation. These results point out an important principle, namely the amount of the drug or dietary supplement is important. If too much is or too little is given these could have negative effects or no effect. The optimum dose is required for the optimum effect.

The important conclusions are that n-3 fatty acids from fish oils lower triglyceride levels both in normal persons and in those with elevated levels of triglycerides. On the other hand the n-6 fatty acids may increase blood levels of triglycerides in some individuals. Dietary n-3 fatty acids from fish have a strong triglyceride-lowering effect. Also important is that elevated levels of blood triglycerides are a new risk factor for CAD.

Dietary saturated triglycerides rich in palmitic and stearic acid tend to increase blood lipid levels. It is clear that to speak only in broad terms of dietary fat or unsaturated fatty acids as a means of regulating blood lipid levels is no longer sufficient. One must specify the type and amount of unsaturated fatty acid and its dietary source. Docosahexenoic acid is important for the function of brain and retina (Connor et al 1992) but also for the heart and nerves. Studies by Willett have shown that DHA and n-3 polyunsaturated fatty acids protect against heart arrhythmias (irregular heart beats).

Effects of Dietary Fats and Obesity on the Level of Blood Lipids

High risk patients should first begin a program of diet and exercise therapy for at least three to six months before starting drug therapy. This includes restriction of foods high in cholesterol and saturated fats, substituting the bad saturated fats with the good n-3 polyunsaturated fats, and restricting total daily calories to prevent overweight. Lean meats such as veal, chicken breast, turkey breast, and fish should replace fatty meats such as hamburgers, sausage, and fatty steaks. The manner in which diet fats and obesity influence plasma lipid levels is shown inTable 2.7 below.

Table 2.7 How Dietary fats and obesity influence blood lipid levels	
Factor	**Effect**
Excess dietary cholesterol	**Suppresses the synthesis of LDL receptors, increases cholesterol level**
Excess dietary saturated fat and trans fat	**Reduces the activity and level of LDL receptors, increases VLDL synthesis, increases the level of cholesterol and triglycerides**
Obesity	**Increases the synthesis of VLDL and IDL and increases the level of cholesterol and triglycerides**

The recommended daily intake of cholesterol in the U.S. is about 300 mg/day. Since one egg has about this amount, this means that one should not eat more than one egg a day. However, as discussed in more detail in chapter 2, there is no compelling evidence supporting this restriction and estimates are that for most persons it is safe to eat three to four eggs a week. Also eating fish and taking fish oil capsules will counter act some of the rise in blood cholesterol from eating eggs.

It is noteworthy that dietary cholesterol and saturated fat decrease the level of LDL receptors and thus elevate blood cholesterol level. LDL receptors are covered in Chapter 7. There may be other effects of saturated and trans fatty acids, including effects on the structure and properties of the lipoproteins, and on the structure and normal function of cell membrane fluidity.

Fish n-3 Fatty Acids Protect Against Heart Attack and Stroke

The information mentioned above becomes more important when one considers the other major effect of n-3 polyunsaturated fatty acids as anticlotting agents. The n-3 fatty acids inhibit platelet aggregation. Fish oil n-3 fatty acids give a longer bleeding time in humans as judged by the Ivy test, in which the bleeding time of a small cut in the skin is measured.

Why is the antithrombic effect of fish oils important? The answer relates to the role of platelets in forming a thrombus (clot) and the role of fatty acids on platelet aggregation. The n-3 fatty acids inhibit platelet aggregation and thus inhibit clots formed by platelets. This protects humans against heart attack and stroke.

Two major factors, atherosclerosis and clot formation, lead to occlusion of arteries and subsequent heart attack or stroke. A coronary artery may be occluded by 50–70 percent without causing a major problem since most coronary arteries have an excess of blood flow. However, if a vessel that is 70–90 percent occluded is then subjected to thrombus formation, a thrombus can immediately shut off all or so much blood flow that this will lead to a heart attack or stroke. Therefore, the intake of n-3 fatty acids not only lowers blood cholesterol levels, which protects from atherosclerosis, but also inhibits thrombus formation that offers protection from heart attack and stroke.

In summary, eating fish in place of beef and pork offers the following health benefits:

1. protection from CAD by lowering the levels of blood cholesterol and triglycerides.

2. protection from cancer.

3. protection from inflammation.

4. protection from thrombosis which cause heart attack and stroke.

5. protection from irregular heart beats (arrhythmias).

Exercise and Heart Disease

Dr. Willett stresses the importance of exercise in protecting persons from heart disease. Population studies show that moderate exercise (such as uninterrupted fast walking for 30 min/day or walking three times a day for ten minutes) offers protection from heart disease and decreases the incidence of mortality. Moderate sustained exercise by walking daily avoids the stress on joints and the heart that can be produced by long jogging.

The beneficial effect of exercise on mortality was demonstrated in studies comparing rural mail clerks with rural delivery mailmen. Mortality was lower in walking mailmen. Studies also show that bus drivers have a much higher incidence of heart attacks than do men in the general population. This increased susceptibility to heart attacks is attributable in part to stress on the job and in part to lack of exercise. Listed below are the benefits of exercise.

1. Prolonged moderate exercise (walking) increases collateral circulation in the heart that provides more blood to the heart.

2. Exercise maintains muscle tone and strengthens bones.

3. Exercise burns off excess fat and excess glucose that lowers the blood sugar level and the blood insulin level. These actions protect against getting type-2 diabetes.

4. Exercise also provides more blood to the brain that may help slow down memory loss.

5. Exercise protects against blood clots from forming in the large veins of the legs (phlebitis). When blood flow is diminished by long periods of sitting down while driving a car or taking a plane ride, this enhances the clot formation. Clots can lead to a heart attack or stroke.

Exercise should be enjoyable. This can be achieved by exercising to music, walking with friends or other persons, and by joining a health club. During hot weather and during very cold weather my wife and I walk inside malls or walk up and down steps in our three level home…

Eating should be enjoyable. However, the hard earned benefits of exercise and dieting are easily reversed by overeating on holidays of which when including birthdays, and graduations, there are many in the U. S. During holidays most persons eat "bad" foods like hot dogs, beef hamburgers, pies, cakes, potato chips, potato salad, ice cream, and drink sodas and beer in excess. Unfortunately overeating these foods cause weight gain which is difficult to undo. Many persons believe that on these days it is ok to break the rules and that they are entitled to some freedom of diets. I do not disagree with this point. However, losing weight is difficult but gaining weight is easy.

The question that often is raised is "Is it worth it to sacrifice the joy of eating on these holidays or other days just to gain a few extra years of life?" The answer to this question is left up to each person. I recall my father often saying he would rather enjoy overeating and sacrifice 5 years of life rather than go on diets. He did this but died of a heart attack at age 72. He was a happy man and lived good life but was willing to risk a shorter life span for the joy of eating. I chose a different course by controlling my food intake, exercising daily, and taking necessary medication. I hope to live a long life.

The next chapter 3 discusses lipid lowering drugs when diets are not successful mainly because of lack of compliance or lack of will to keep on diets. Readers who are interested in the biochemical aspects of lipids can refer to chapter 5 for the metabolism of fatty acids, chapter 6 for the metabolism of cholesterol, and chapter 7 for the metabolism of blood lipoproteins.

Chapter 3

Drug Therapies for High Levels of Blood Lipids and Treatment of Blood Clots

Lipid-Lowering Drugs

Dietary management and exercise should be tried first for a period of 3 to 6 months to lower blood levels of cholesterol and triglycerides in patients having high blood lipids before drug therapy is used. Many patients find it difficult to be on a restricted and regimented diet for a long period of time. Hence compliance to diets is compromised. In this situation, drug therapy is necessary to maintain blood lipid levels in the normal range. The current lipid lowering drugs are shown in the table below in Table 3.1.

Table 3.1 Lipid lowering Drugs

Mevacor (lovastatin, mevinolin)
Pravachol (pravastatin)
Zocor (simvastatin)
Lipitor (atorvastatin)
Lescol (fluvastatin)
Baycol (cerivastatin) no longer in use
Vytorin (simvastatin plus ezetimbe)
Crestor (rosuvastatin)
Lopid (Gemfibrizol, Atromid-S
Colestid (Questran, Cholestryamine)
Probucol (Lorelco)
Niacin (Nicotinic acid)
Plant sterols (sitosterol, ergosterol)

The statin drugs work by inhibiting the rate limiting enzyme reaction in the synthesis of cholesterol. This enzyme is HMG-CoA reductase (HMGR). The statins are Mevacor, Pravachol, Lescol, Baychol, Lipitor, Zocor, Crestor, and Vytorin. Vytorin contains a statin and ezetimbe which is a synthetic sterol that inhibits the absorption of cholesterol.

The drugs used for patients with high levels of both cholesterol and triglycerides (i.e. blood cholesterol level > 230 mg/dl and triglyceride level >250 mg/dl) are a statin plus Colestid. The statin drugs inhibit the synthesis of cholesterol and have a greater effect in lowering blood cholesterol than lowering blood triglycerides.

Other drugs used to lower blood lipids include Niacin (nicotinic acid), Lopid (Atromid-S, or Gemfibrizol), Probucol (Lorelco), and certain plant sterols (sitosterol, ergosterol).

Recently some plant sterols and synthetic sterols have been made available to the public as substitutes for the Statins and other prescription drugs. Long term controlled clinical studies on humans have yet to be done on the benefit of these sterols. Plant sterols inhibit the absorption of cholesterol in the intestines. Since the liver makes all the cholesterol the body needs it is not apparent how just inhibiting cholesterol absorption alone can decrease enough the blood cholesterol level. This may be why Vytorin has both a statin and a synthetic sterol.

The plant sterols apparently are not absorbed by the body and thus it appears that they should not exert an inhibitory effect on cholesterol synthesis in the liver or on the LDL receptor. The full mechanism of action of plant sterols remains to be determined. The plant sterols do act as a drain on cholesterol from the blood by preventing the absorption of cholesterol in the intestines and allowing the cholesterol to be lost in the feces. In his respect the plant sterols act like Colestid which binds bile acids. Colestid alone does not give a very large decrease in blood cholesterol. For this reason, Colestid is used in combination with a statin drug.

Colestid is a resin polymer that binds bile acids in the intestines and drains cholesterol from the body. This forces the liver to convert more cholesterol to bile acids and thus the cholesterol level in the blood decreases. However, in my experience, Colestid alone has little effect on blood triglyceride level and only a modest effect on lowering blood cholesterol. Patients who have normal cholesterol levels but have a high triglyceride level can be treated with Niacin (nicotinic acid) or Lopid (also known as Atromid-S or Gemfibrizol) **but they must avoid taking a statin with these drugs.**

Colestid has been used for patients with elevated plasma cholesterol. This insoluble polymer drug is taken suspended in fruit juices or water. The dose varies from 10 to 30 g/day, depending on the degree of hypercholesterolemia and the dosage that the patient can tolerate. They reduce plasma cholesterol (mainly LDL-cholesterol) by 13–25 percent. Patient compliance with these bile acid-binding resins has been low. Constipation, especially at higher doses, is an undesirable side effect. Because of these side effects, the use of Colestid has decreased and is replaced by one of the Statins.

The Statins are recommended for patients with elevated cholesterol, especially LDL-cholesterol. Taken in doses of 10–40 mg per day, these drugs lower cholesterol (mainly LDL-cholesterol by 30–60 percent and increases HDL-cholesterol by 8–11 percent. Probucol (Lorelco) lowers plasma cholesterol. Probucol does not lower plasma triglycerides but unfortunately may decrease plasma HDL levels.

All of the drugs may affect the liver (and other organs) and increase the level of certain liver enzymes such as alkaline phosphatase and transaminase enzymes in plasma. Therefore, all patients need to be monitored on a routine basis. The very long-term effects (over a period of 40 years) of these drugs have not been determined. Cholestryamine and Niacin have been in use for many years, whereas Mevacor has been available as a prescription drug only since 1987 and the newer Statins have been in use for a much shorter time.

The costs of these lipid-lowering drugs vary widely. At present, the most expensive drugs are the Statins and the least expensive drug is niacin. Slow-release niacin pills are now available but cost more than regular niacin. The monthly costs of these drugs can vary from as little as $2.00 for niacin (1 g/day dose) to over $100 for a Statin, (20 mg per day).

The normal and abnormal values for blood total cholesterol, LDL cholesterol and HDL cholesterol are shown in Table 3.2 below. These values change with time as new information is obtained from clinical studies.

Table 3.2 Normal and abnormal values of blood cholesterol (mg/dL)				
Lipid	Normal range	Borderline high	High	Very high
Cholesterol (total)	< 200	200–239	> 240	> 300
LDL cholesterol	100–129	130–159	160–189	> 190
HDL cholesterol For men	40–50	NA*	NA	NA
HDL cholesterol, For women	50–90	NA	NA	NA

*NA= non applicable. The values are estimates and vary in different laboratories and with time as new knowledge is obtained. The results are based on fasting blood samples but the analyses are done of plasma obtained from blood. Note that high levels of LDL have a high risk for heart disease and high values of HDL have a low risk for heart disease. A desirable LDL/HDL ratio should be 3 or less.

High Levels of Blood Triglycerides: A New Risk Factor for Heart Disease)

Recent analyses of prospective studies indicate that elevated triglycerides are also an independent risk factor for CAD. Factors that increase triglycerides are obesity and overweight, lack of physical exercise, cigarette smoking, excess alcohol intake, high carbohydrate and high lipid diets, and several diseases (diabetes, renal failure, nephritic syndrome), and certain drugs (corticosteroids, estrogen, retinoids, high doses of beta-adrenergic antagonists), and genetic disorders.

Patients with very high triglyceride levels may need to be put on diets with triglycerides having medium chain fatty acids (MCT) plus drug therapy. MCTs have fatty acids with less than 12 carbon atoms. The digestion of MCT is rapid and complete. Gastric lipases hydrolyze MCT and the released fatty acids can be absorbed in part through the stomach into the portal vein.

The medium chain fatty acids have increased solubility compared to long-chain fatty acids and bypass the conversion to fattyacylCoAs. This enables the fatty acids to encounter the liver first where they undergo beta oxidation without the need of being transported by the carnitine cycle. This leads to more pronounced production of ketones. MCTs have been used for patients with pancreatitis, bilary insufficiency, gastroenteritis, obesity, diabetes, and for parenteral nutrition.

Niacin in doses of 1–6 g/day may be used for patients with elevated plasma triglycerides. (It is noteworthy that niacinamide, the amide form of niacin, is not effective). Niacin reduces plasma triglyceride by about 9–20 percent. Starting the patient with a low dose (100 mg/day) and increasing the dosage over a period of 1–2 weeks prevents the severe flushing that initially may occur. Giving aspirin during this initial period also helps prevent flushing. Lopid doses of 0.6–3 g/day may be used for patients with elevated triglycerides. It lowers plasma cholesterol by 2–9 percent.

The Statins are recommended for patients with elevated cholesterol, especially LDL-cholesterol. Taken in doses of 10–40 mg per day, the Statin drugs lower cholesterol (mainly LDL-cholesterol by 30–60 percent and increases HDL-cholesterol by 8–11 percent.

All of the drugs may have hepatic effects that lead to increases in certain liver enzymes such as alkaline phosphatase and transaminases in plasma. Therefore, all patients need to be carefully monitored. The very long-term effects (over a period of 30–40 years) of these drugs have not been determined. The first statin drug Mevacor has been available as a prescription drug about the early 1980s.

The costs of these lipid-lowering drugs vary widely. At present, the most expensive drugs are the Statins and the least expensive drug is niacin. Colestid and Lopid are less expensive than the Statins but more expensive than niacin. Slow-release Niacin pills are now available and cost more than regular Niacin. Thus, the monthly costs of these drugs can vary from as little as $2.00 for Niacin (1 g/day dose) to over $100 for a Statin, (10 to 20 mg per day).

Studies on Blood Triglycerides)

For a long time triglyceride levels in blood were not regarded as a risk factor for heart disease. However, recent prospective studies indicate that elevated triglycerides are also an independent risk factor for CAD. Factors that increase triglycerides include obesity and overweight, lack of physical exercise, cigarette smoking, excess alcohol intake, high carbohydrate and high lipid diets, and several diseases (diabetes, renal failure, nephritic syndrome. Some drugs also increase blood triglyceride levels ((corticosteroids, estrogen, retinoids, and high doses of beta-adrenergic antagonists). Normal and abnormal levels of blood triglycerides are shown in Table 3.3 below.

Table 3.3 Normal and abnormal levels of blood triglycerides	
Normal triglycerides	< 150 mg/dl
Borderline high	150–199 mg/dl
High	200–499 mg/dl
Very high	> 500 mg/dl

Combined Drug Therapy

More dramatic effects in lowering plasma cholesterol levels in humans have been achieved by using a combination of two drugs. The combinations that have been tried are Colestid plus Niacin, Colestid plus Lopid, or Colestid plus a Statin.

The new statin drug Vytorin has both a Statin and a synthetic sterol that inhibits cholesterol absorption. This combination may reduce blood cholesterol somewhat more than other statins. A combination of drugs may be more effective than either drug alone because the drugs act at different points in cholesterol metabolism. Indeed, whereas each drug alone may give a reduction of plasma cholesterol about 10–30 percent, the combination of drugs lowers plasma cholesterol by 40–60 percent. Thus the statin drugs inhibit the synthesis of cholesterol whereas Colestid inhibits the absorption of cholesterol. This dual action is very effective in lowering blood cholesterol levels.

The actual amount of reduction depends on the dose of each drug and on patient compliance in taking the drugs. Diets low in cholesterol, low in saturated and trans fats but high in n-3 fatty acids augment the effectiveness of the drugs. On the other hand, patients feel that they can indulge in food because they are on medication. This is counterproductive since it will lessen the effectiveness of the lipid-lowering drugs.

The statin drugs should not be used in combination with Niacin or Lopid since together they can cause severe muscle damage or kidney damage (rhabdomyolysis) and death. This occurred with a few patients who were given the new statin Baychol plus niacin or Lopid and may occur with combinations of niacin or Lopid with any statin drug. Baychol was removed from the market in 2001.

Clinical Trials with Lipid Lowering Drugs

The CLAS (cholesterol-lowering atherosclerosis) study was a randomized, placebo-controlled, angiographic trial testing Colestid (30 g/day) and niacin (3–12 g/day) therapy in 162 nonsmoking men ages 40–59 years with previous coronary bypass surgery. During the 2 years of treatment there was a 26 percent reduction in total plasma cholesterol, a 43 percent reduction in LDL-cholesterol, and a simultaneous elevation of HDL-cholesterol.

This resulted in a significant reduction in the average number of atherosclerotic lesions (atheromas) in the coronary arteries per subject. Also, the percentage of subjects with new lesions or adverse change in the coronary artery bypass graphs was significantly reduced.

Deterioration in overall coronary status was significantly less in drug-treated subjects. Regression of atherosclerosis, as indicated by improvement in overall coronary status, occurred in 16.2 percent of Colestid-Niacin-treated subjects versus 2.4 percent in the placebo group (Blankenhorn et al., 1987). This study shows that plaque regression can occur and gives hope that further studies will provide more information on how to speed up plaque regression.

Pravachol and Lipitor were investigated in the "PROVE IT" study in 2002 by Bristol Myers. The results presented at the *American College of Cardiology* meetings in 2004 showed that taking Lipitor gave a 16 percent lower risk of heart attacks or death than those taking Pravachol. The sales of the Statin drugs are now in the billions of dollars per year in the US.

It is noteworthy that the drug actions described above apply to heterozygous type 2 hyperlipoproteinemia (familial hypercholesterolemia) since people with this condition have only one defective gene for the LDL receptor and their cholesterol levels can be reduced from high values of 300–400 mg/dl to values of 150–200 mg/dl.

However, people who are homozygous for type 2 hyperlipoproteinemia, have cholesterol levels of 800–1200 mg/dl; since they have inherited two defective genes for the LDL receptor, drug therapy is not effective since even with drug therapy these individuals may have cholesterol levels 400 mg/dl or higher. These patients have very little or no LDL receptors and are refractory to drug therapy and need a liver transplant.

Persons with type 3 and 4 hyperlipoproteinemia can be treated effectively with drug therapy since they have normal LDL receptors and can reduce their elevated plasma cholesterol levels from high values of 280–350 mg/dl to a normal range of 150–200 mg/dl, especially when drug therapy is administered in conjunction with dietary management and exercise.

Fake Drugs, a Pending Crisis in the U.S.

The public is now on notice that many fake drugs are on the market in the U.S. and Europe. The fake drugs and their labeling look very much like the authentic drugs. The popular drugs such as Lipitor, Viagra, Advil, Levitra, and many others are now being made in China, Mexico, and Central America. Some of these drugs have now entered some well-known drug stores and in a few cases has led to death of innocent persons. The pharmaceutical companies and the FDA must use all their power and knowledge to counteract these fraud drugs for the safety of the American public. If fraud drugs are not stopped, the U.S. will face a huge health crisis.

Stopping fraud drugs may be done by frequently changing the size, shape, and color of the drug and putting a very small amount of an inert substance which can easily be detected. The labeling of the drugs and the shape and size of the bottles may also can be modified at frequent intervals. The use of some hard to produce magnetic bar codes may be developed. Otherwise the pharmacies have to develop detecting systems to monitor all the drugs they get from their distributors. The pharmaceutical salesmen and women could have hard to fake identifications to assure the pharmacies that they are authentic representatives.

Platelet Aggregation Forms a Platelet Clot (Thrombus).

I believe it is important for persons to have some knowledge of blood clots because blood clots cause heart attacks and stroke.

Hemostasis is the stopping of bleeding caused by injury to the blood vessels. The first phase is constriction of the injured vessels to slow down the bleeding. The second phase consists of the formation of a platelet plug (white thrombus) at the injured site. The third phase is the formation of a red thrombus (blood clot) resulting from red cells being trapped in the platelet plug. The fourth phase is the dissolution of the clot. Blood clotting and dissolution are believed to occur frequently in the body without causing symptoms.

Platelet aggregation occurs when platelets bind to collagen in arteries. This binding makes the platelets aggregate, change shape, become sticky and form a thrombus (clot). Clot formation in the blood can cause a heart attack, stroke and emphysema. A blood clot can be formed by blood platelets or blood fibrin.

Thrombin Converts Fibrinogen to Fibrin Clots.

The enzyme thrombin is generated from prothrombin when tissue thromboplastin is released from injured cells. Thromboplastin converts inactive prothrombin to active thrombin. Thrombin converts fibrinogen to fibrin that forms a fibrin clot that stops the bleeding.

Drugs Used to Treat Blood Clots

Fibrinolysis is the dissolution of the fibrin clot. When fibrin forms, it binds plasminogen that activates tissue plasminogen activator (TPA). TPA stimulates the conversion of plasminogen to plasmin at the site of injury. Plasmin digests fibrin and fibrinogen and dissolves the clot.

Streptokinase or TPA is used to treat patients who are having a heart attack or stroke. They form a complex with plasminogen and in the process convert inactive plasminogen to active plasmin. When streptokinase is infused into a patient, a sufficient amount must be used to overcome circulating antistreptococcal antibodies and antiplasmin. Care must be taken because excessive fibrinolysis can lead to serious bleeding problems. TPA must be used for stroke victims within 3 to 4 hours of onset of symptoms that include blurred vision, weakness in one or both arms or legs, slurred speech, crooked smile, and difficulty in maintaining balance when walking.

The Second International Study of Infarct Survival, involving about 17,000 patients showed that streptokinase or aspirin alone reduced mortality caused by a heart attack by about 25 percent, but when the two agents were given together they reduced mortality by more than 40 percent. Both drugs are most effective within 4 hours of onset of chest pain. Newer forms of both TPA and streptokinase are being developed that hopefully will have less side effects and be more effective than the current drugs.

Other drugs that inhibit clot formation are the nonsteroidal antiinflammatory agents, thromboxane synthetase inhibitors (dipyridamole) and cyclooxygenase inhibitors (Celebrex, and aspirin).

Aspirin Therapy to Prevent Blood Clots From Platelets.

The common drug that provides protection against heart attack and stroke caused by a clot or thrombus is aspirin (acetylsalicylic acid). Indeed, only one baby aspirin (81 mg) per day is effective. It is unfortunate that the price of the smaller 81 mg aspirin pill is higher than the price of the larger 325 mg aspirin pill. The 81 mg pill of aspirin inhibits nearly completely platelet aggregation by thromboxaneTXA_2. Some doctors still prefer to use the 325 mg aspirin for patients who have had coronary artery disease.

Numerous studies have been done on the effectiveness of aspirin in protecting humans from heart attacks and strokes. Initial studies yielded mixed results because of the different dosages used (one to four aspirin tablets, equivalent to 325–1300 mg per day). A dose of one to three aspirin tablets per day is commonly used to treat men in the very early stage of a heart attack or a mini stroke (caused by a clot). This treatment may provide a 40 percent reduction in stroke occurrence in men but has been less effective in women.

A British study found a 25 percent reduction in recurrent heart attacks among patients taking one aspirin pill (325 mg) a day. In seven studies done in the United States, Canada and Europe five indicated favorable results and three gave equivocal results based on mortality rate and number of nonfatal heart attacks. Recently however, a study (Young et al., 1988) by Harvard University on 22,071 male physicians has shown that taking one aspirin every other day provides 40 percent protection against fatal heart attack. It is hoped that a similar protection will be found in women.

Like any drug, aspirin has side effects in some humans. In particular, some young children may be more susceptible to Reye's syndrome when they take aspirin. Aspirin also can aggravate symptoms associated with peptic ulcers. Slow release aspirin (coated aspirin) is available and recommended since it reduces the adverse effects of aspirin on bleeding in the stomach or intestines. Aspirin therapy is not used for patients who may be having or who have had a bleeding stroke.

Prostaglandins and the Enzymes COX 1 and COX 2

The eicosanoids consist of the prostaglandins, thrombaxanes, lipoxins, and leukotrienes. The prostaglandins and thromboxanes are called prostanoids. Prostaglandins are made by the prostate gland, thromboxanes are made by platelets (also called thrombocytes), and leukotrienes are made by white blood cells (leukocytes).

The main eicosanoids are derived from the n-6 fatty acid arachidonic acid, which has four double bonds. Minor eicosanoids are made from the n-3 eicosapentenoic acid, which has five double bonds. All mammalian cells except red blood cells can synthesize eicosanoids. These important biological molecules have profound physiological effects at very low concentrations (in the micromolar or picomolar range).

The non-steroidal anti-infammatory drugs (NSAIDs) consist of ibuprofen (found in Advil and Alleve), Naproxen, indomethacin, phenylbutazone, and aspirin. All these drugs inhibit the COX-1 and COX-2 enzymes. Because the inhibition of COX-1 in the stomach and intestines is associated with NSAID induced ulcers, pharmaceutical companies have developed drugs targeted more specifically against COX-2, an inducible enzyme, whose level in cells can increase and cause undesirable side effects. The drugs acting as inhibitors of COX-2 include Celebrex and Prexige.

Recently the COX-2 inhibitory drugs Vioxx and Bextra have been recalled because reports show that they can increase the incidence of heart attacks and stroke in some patients.

The corticosteroids (like prednisone) inhibit phospholipase A_2. This inhibits the release of arachidonic acid, the precursor of the prostaglandins. Corticosteroids are thus effective in treating inflammatory conditions such as joint pain in arthritis, and muscle pain but their dose should be kept as low as possible. Over a long time use they can have serious side effects.

Drug Dosage:

The dose of any drug has to consider the weight, sex, age, and health condition of the patient. Smaller lower weight persons have a smaller blood volume and consequently require a lower dose of the drug. Older persons may not metabolize the drug as fast as younger persons and may require a smaller dose of the drug. Alcoholics may have hyperplasia of the liver endoplasmic reticulum that detoxifies the drugs and hence they are more refractory to the drugs as compared to persons who do not consume much alcohol.

How the sex of a person influences the dose of a drug needs to be more fully studied. The goal is to use the smallest amount of the drug that is effective in treating the particular disease thereby minimizing the toxic side effects of the drug. Nearly all drugs may have toxic or undesirable side effects but fortunately only a very small number of persons have these side effects.

Drugs given orally are absorbed mainly from the intestines and then go directly to the liver where they are detoxified. On the other hand drugs given intravenously got directly into the blood and are dispersed over the entire body and do not go directly into the liver. The absorption of drugs by the intestines is influenced by the types of foods a person eats, how much water the person drinks and the calcium and iron content of the water.

The drug enters the blood and reaches a maximum high value and then the drug concentration declines slowly over time. The peak concentration may vary from 1 to several hours. Drugs that can be given by patch are slowly absorbed and this allows for a more steady and prolonged blood concentration of the drug. Newer methods for drug delivery using computer controlled pumps are now available in limited cases such as the delivery of insulin for diabetics.

Drugs also vary in their solubility and this influences how fast they are absorbed into the body whether they are given orally or by patch. Some drugs may form insoluble complexes with calcium and iron in the foods that are consumed at the same time. This will decrease the absorption of the drug.

The storage of the drugs is important. Humidity, light, and heat can degrade the drug. Drugs must be protected from the humidity of bath rooms and the heat from stoves and from bright lighted areas. All drugs should show the time of expiration of the drug as well as their major side effects and dose. The drugs do not suddenly expire on the expiration day. After the expiration date, the drug may remain active from 3 months to possibly one year and undergo a slow loss of potency. It is advisable to check with the drug company for more details on this matter.

Each prescription drug comes with a vast amount of information on the drugs properties, metabolism, excretion, etc. and on side effects including tables, which much of the public may not fully understand. For most patients it would be desirable to have a simplified sheet of information stressing how much drug to take, how often, and the major side effects in large print that is easy to read.

Effects of Excess Alcohol Intake on Health

Estimate show that the average adult American consumes about 3 gallons of alcohol per year and that approximately 10 million Americans are alcoholics. About 3 million teenagers in the United States drink in excess. Alcohol-related deaths in the United States number close to 150,000 per year. The average adult American consumes about 3 gallons of alcohol per year and that approximately 10 million Americans are alcoholics. About 3 million teenagers in the United States drink in excess. Alcohol-related deaths in the United States number close to 150,000 per year.

Alcohol abuse costs the United States about $50 billion per year due to loss of work, health costs, motor accidents, and fire loss. Fifty percent of highway fatalities are attributed to excessive alcohol consumption. Excessive drinking of alcohol kills more young persons than does taking hard drugs.

Alcohol affects all organs of the body. Excessive alcohol intake inhibits protein synthesis in liver, heart, and muscle and can cause heart enlargement, muscle weakness, fatty liver, alcoholic hepatitis, liver cirrhosis, hypoglycemia, ketoacidosis, coma, ascites (fluid accumulation in the abdomen), and esophageal swollen veins which can rupture and cause death by uncontrolled bleeding. Failure of the liver to produce clotting proteins aggravates the bleeding.

Excessive intake of alcohol also leads to malnutrition and vitamin deficiencies. A deficiency of vitamin B-12 and folic acid can lead to anemia. Alcohol intake inhibits fetal growth, especially in the last trimester, and can lead to brain damage. This abnormality is known as fetal alcohol syndrome.

Ethanol (CH_3CH_2OH) is also called ethyl alcohol or simply alcohol by most clinicians. The oxidation of 1 g of ethanol in the body to carbon dioxide and water yields 7 kcal of energy and produces 0.9 g of water. The biochemical and clinical effects of excessive intake of alcohol will be considered.

Metabolism of Alcohol

Alcohol is oxidized primarily in the liver in a two step shown below in Figure 3.1.

Figure 3.1 Oxidation of alcohol by enzymes

Step 1 Alcohol + NAD ———> Acetaldehyde + NADH

Step 2 Acetaldehyde + NAD ——> Acetic acid + NADH

Step 1 is uses the enzyme alcohol dehydrogenase (ADH) and requires the coenzyme NAD^+ whereas Step 2 uses the enzyme aldehyde dehydrogenase (ALDH) and also requires NAD^+. Thus, the oxidation of 1 mole of ethanol to acetate produces 2 moles of NADH, and this increases very markedly the $NADH/NAD^+$ ratio in the liver cell. This high ratio inhibits glucose formation causing low blood sugar, but increases the synthesis of fatty acids and triglycerides.

Alcohol Effects on the Heart

Alcohol taken in excess affects cellular substructures in the heart. Mitochondrial respiration and calcium uptake are inhibited. Acetaldehyde has a direct effect on heart protein synthesis. Malfunction of the heart muscle is revealed by disturbances in calcium uptake.

Acetaldehyde is a direct vasodilator in the heart. It has a stronger action in stimulating the release of norepinephrine at nerve terminals, which leads to vasoconstriction and increased blood pressure. This in turn leads to hypertension (high blood pressure) and bradycardia (rapid heart rate).

Moderate intake of alcohol (one or two glasses of wine per day) increases only modestly, the level of HDL in the blood. Whether the modest increase in HDL offers protection from the risk of coronary heart disease is not known with certainty. Even a modest amount of alcohol intake increases the synthesis of VLDL in liver and hence increases the level of VLDL triglycerides in plasma an effect that may be deleterious to persons having genetic induced hyperlipidemia. Therefore, this potential beneficial effect of alcohol intake varies, depending on each person's genetic make-up and ability to synthesize and degrade plasma lipoproteins.

Alcohol Effects on the Action of Drugs

The increased gastric blood flow resulting from alcohol intake, coupled with the solvency of alcohol, can produce increased rates of drug absorption and heightened drug effects. When taken as a single large dose, alcohol inhibits the drug detoxifying enzymes in the liver and makes a person more sensitive to (less tolerant of) the action of the drug. This effect is mediated by an inhibition of the detoxifying enzymes in liver.

However, chronic intake (long term) of alcohol leads to hyperplasia (increased growth) of the endoplasmic reticulum and hence increased levels of the detoxifying enzymes and therefore makes a person more resistant (more tolerant) to the action of the drugs.

The next chapter covers the history and epidemiologic studies done on atherosclerosis as related to CAD. Readers interested in cholesterol metabolism and in blood lipoproteins can refer to chapter 6 and chapter 7.

Chapter 4

Atherosclerosis and Coronary Artery Disease (CAD)

Atherosclerosis (the development of lipid plaques in arteries) is a major health problem in the United States. Atherosclerosis is the accumulation of lipid-rich plaques on the inner lining (intima) of arteries of the body. Advanced plaques are the result of an accumulation of cholesterol, cholesterol esters, phospholipids, live and dead cells, calcium, and other components including collagen, elastin, and proteoglycans. Plaques can be large enough to severely restrict the flow of blood to tissues or can narrow the lumen of arteries to a degree that enhances formation of a thrombus that plugs the artery and leads to a coronary heart attack or to a stroke.

Heart diseases rank number 1 and cerebrovascular diseases (includes strokes) rank number 3 with respect to the number of deaths per 100,000 persons. The causes of death in the US are shown below in Table 4.1.

Table 4.1 Causes of Death in the U.S.*	
Cause of death	**Deaths per 100,000**
Heart disease	324
Malignant neoplasms (cancer)	192
Cerebrovascular diseases	66
Unintentional injuries	40
Chronic obstructive pulmonary disease	29
Pneumonia, influenza	25
Suicide, homicide	21
Diabetes	16
Chronic liver disease, cirrhosis	11
Congenital anomalies	6
Prematurity	4
Sudden infant death syndrome	2

*From the Center for Disease Control 1986, and from Marinetti, G.V. 1990 Chapter 6, Table 6-1, page 122 with kind permission from Springer Science and Business Media. Values are rounded to the nearest whole number.

Cerebrovascular diseases (stroke and blood vessel disease) are related to atherosclerosis, abnormal lipid metabolism, and platelet aggregation. Traits that may predict the occurrence of coronary heart disease (CHD) are called risk factors. Coronary heart disease (CHD) is now called by the more specific term coronary artery disease (CAD). A risk factor is correlated with the probability that a given individual will develop a disease. Risk factors are usually identified in prospective studies in a large population by observing the correlation between the putative risk factor and the occurrence of the disease.

Risk factors are not always a direct cause of the disease. Moreover, their absence does not indicate that the disease will not occur. The probability of developing CAD increases with the number and severity of the positive risk factors in a given individual. The three primary risk factors for CAD and stroke are high blood pressure (systolic pressure >140 mm Hg and diastolic pressure >90 mm Hg), elevated blood cholesterol (especially a high LDL-cholesterol and a low HDL-cholesterol), and smoking. The risk factors for CAD are shown below in Table 4.2.

Table 4.2 Risk factors for coronary artery disease (CAD)*	
Modifiable	**Fixed**
Hypercholesterolemia	Genetic mutations
Hypertension	Age
Smoking	Sex (male)
Diabetes mellitus	Family history of CAD
Low HDL cholesterol < 35 mg/dl	
High LDL cholesterol > 160 mg/dl	
Obesity (30% overweight)	
Personality type A	
Stress	

*From Marinetti, G.V., 1990 Chapter 6, Table 6-1, page 122 with kind permission of Springer Science and Business Media.

Overweight (obesity), diabetes, sex, age, and personality type are secondary risk factors. However CAD can occur without known risk factors. Persons with Friedman type A personality appear to be at higher risk for heart disease. Type A personality is characterized by impatience, urge to meet deadlines, hostility toward others, and tendency to become readily angered or excited by trivial matters. Stress is now considered a risk factor that promotes disease by increasing blood pressure and by altering the stress hormones in the body.

Although elevated levels of hormones such as epinephrine, testosterone, and ACTH may be links between type A personality and CAD, these links are not well defined. Platelet aggregation and high blood pressure, which are exacerbated by elevated levels of epinephrine, may be one link. Whether type A personality is a risk factor for CAD is still controversial.

Atherosclerosis affects millions of humans. The disease can begin early in life, is usually a very slow process, and predisposes one to developing CAD. In 1986 about 200,000 coronary artery bypass operations were done in the United States. This number rose to about 250,000 in 1988 and has increased in the subsequent years. The medical costs are very high and represent several billion dollars of health expense to the nation. **With the use of stents, diet, exercise, and drug therapy, the number of open heart surgeries has decreased and the number of deaths from heart disease is declining.**

An understanding of the process of atherogenesis is vital to effective treatment of heart disease and stroke. The relationship between elevated plasma cholesterol levels (especially LDL cholesterol) and the risk of atherosclerosis and CAD has been substantiated by a number of studies on laboratory animals, epidemiological studies between and within human populations, genetic studies, and clinical trials.

Early History of Atherosclerosis

Aortas of Egyptian mummies showed the presence of atherosclerotic plaques. The plaques were called atheroma from the Greek athere (mush). In 1818, Chevruel identified cholesterol in human bile and named it from the Greek chole (bile) and steros (solid). Vogel identified cholesterol in plaques in 1843. In the 1950s, Berchow, Duguid, French, Packman, and Mustard helped develop the response to injury hypothesis to explain plaque formation. In 1900, Windaus found that plaques contained 7 times the amount of cholesterol and 25 times as much cholesterol ester as did normal arteries. The thrombogenic theory of atherogenesis was proposed by Rokitansky in 1952, when the role of platelets in thrombus formation became known.

Experimental Atherosclerosis

Animals develop atherosclerosis when fed diets that raise plasma cholesterol levels. In 1913 the Russians Ignatowski and Anitschkow fed rabbits diets very high in cholesterol. The rabbits developed plaques very similar to those found in humans. Since then, numerous studies involving feeding of cholesterol-rich diets have been carried out in pigs, chickens, dogs, and monkeys. All of these studies showed that high-cholesterol diets lead to atherosclerosis.

A major question is whether atherosclerosis is a reversible process. It now appears quite clear from both animal and human studies that atherosclerotic lesions undergo slow regression when plasma cholesterol levels are reduced below 190 mg/dl in humans by combined therapy with drugs, diet, and exercise, and by cessation of smoking.

Epidemiological Data

Population studies have shown that persons on low-fat diets have less CAD than do those on high-fat diets, especially diets high in saturated fats, trans fats, and cholesterol. South African Bantus eat very low fat diets and are active physically. They have a mean plasma cholesterol level of 160 mg/dl, and have a very low incidence of CAD. Yemenite Jews and Japanese who migrate to the United States initially have a lower incidence of CAD but eventually after adopting American diets they develop CAD at the same rate as do Americans. During WWI the incidence of heart disease fell in large part as a result of the shortage of food and the decrease in obesity and in lower blood lipids.

The lipid content of human aortic intima increases with age. In particular cholesterol esters derived mainly from LDL accumulate in the intima of arteries with age. Studies have shown that damaged arterial cells take up LDL more rapidly than do normal cells due in large part to the infiltration of the intima with medial smooth muscle cells, monocytes, and macrophages.

A large body of epidemiologic data, including comparisons between various populations throughout the world, supports a direct relationship between plasma cholesterol levels and the rate of development of atherosclerosis and CAD. Premature CAD can result from high plasma cholesterol levels even in the absence of other risk factors.

This is clearly demonstrated in children who have the rare homozygous familial hypercholesterolemia type 2. These children have mutated receptors that do not allow LDL in the blood to be taken up by cells. This defect leads to very high levels of LDL with severe hypercholestrolemia. Cholesterol levels in the plasma of these children are in the 1000–1300 mg/dl range, rather than in the normal range of 140–190 mg/dl. These children develop atherosclerosis and severe CAD very early in life (by age 4–6) and can be helped only by liver and heart transplantation or possibly in the future by stem cell research.

Survey Studies: Cholesterol and Coronary Heart Disease CAD

Large surveys have revealed a positive correlation between level of plasma cholesterol and risk of CAD. This correlation is attributable to the athero-genic effect of elevated plasma levels of cholesterol as illustrated in prospective autopsy studies showing a linear correlation between the concentration of plasma cholesterol and the severity of atherosclerosis.

Several surveys, such as the Framingham Heart Study, the Pooling Project (Anderson et al (1987, Castelli et al (1986) and the Israeli prospective study, all confirm that plasma cholesterol level is correlated significantly with the prevalence of CAD.

The MRFIT study involved 356,222 men who were 35–57 years old. They were followed for 6 years and the number of deaths caused by CAD was correlated with their plasma cholesterol level. The relationship was positive throughout and curvilinear. At higher levels of plasma cholesterol (>250 mg/dl) mortality increased more rapidly. The magnitude of the increased risk was fourfold in the top 10 percent as compared with the bottom 10 percent.

A difficulty in demonstrating a correlation between total plasma cholesterol and risk of CAD with values below the mean for any population relates to the opposing effects of cholesterol carried by LDL and HDL. The risk of CAD increases as the level of LDL-cholesterol increases (especially to >150 mg/dl), but the risk falls as the level of HDL-cholesterol increases (especially to >40 mg/dl).

The role of HDL in protecting persons from premature CAD is receiving considerable attention today. The first report from the Framingham study that demonstrated an inverse relationship between HDL-cholesterol and incidence of CAD was based on 4 years of surveillance. The subjects, ages 49–82, were followed for 12 years. Participants at the 80th percentile of HDL-cholesterol were found to have half the risk of developing CAD when compared with subjects at the 20th percentile of HDL-cholesterol (Castelli et al., 1986). Indeed, subjects who had HDL-cholesterol levels above 60 mg/dl had less risk of developing CAD even when their total cholesterol levels varied from 200 mg/dl to 260 mg/dl.

The relationship between smoking, high cholesterol levels and CAD is illustrated by data from the MRFIT study. Although the risk ratios at different cholesterol levels are similar for each group, the absolute differences in risk are much higher for smokers.

Because of the positive correlation between plasma cholesterol level and risk of CAD, many investigators believe that the average cholesterol level for the whole population should be lowered as more data is obtained. The question of what constitutes an ideal plasma cholesterol level was addressed by a group of epidemiologists, clinical investigators, and experimental pathologists. They proposed that the ideal cholesterol levels for adults be set at 130–190 mg/dl. **For the sake of simpli-**

fication and reality, the ideal cholesterol level was recommended not to exceed 190 mg/dl. Since cholesterol is needed to make cell membranes, steroid hormones and bile acids, care should be use not to get the cholesterol level too low.

Alcohol Intake and CAD

Modest intake of alcohol (one 6 or 8 ounce glass of wine per day) has been shown to increase modestly the level of plasma HDL. The association between alcohol intake and risk of CAD is U shaped with both nondrinkers and heavy drinkers having a higher incidence of CAD than moderate users of alcohol. The mechanism whereby alcohol intake increases plasma HDL and offers some protection against CAD is not understood. A recent study has shown that moderate intake of alcohol increases the synthesis of HDL and apoA-I in liver. Since apoA-I is a major protein of HDL, this finding explains in part the modest rise in plasma HDL in persons who drink modest amounts of alcohol.

Alcohol influences membrane fluidity. Part of the action of alcohol may be mediated by a fluidity change that increases the functioning of the LDL receptors. Alcohol may also influence the structure of the lipoproteins, which in turn may affect their interaction with membrane receptors that mediate lipoprotein uptake by cells. These are provisional ideas that need further study.

Alcohol intake leads to an increase in plasma triglycerides, primarily as VLDL. Elevated levels of plasma triglycerides are an independent risk factor for CAD (Castelli, 1986), especially in women and in men with HDL levels below 40 mg/dl.

Postulated Mechanisms of Atherosclerosis

The average adult human heart beats about 70 times per minute and pumps approximately 4000 gallons of blood per day through about 60,000 miles of blood vessels. It is estimated that the daily work load of the heart can lift a man to the top of the Empire State Building. The constant pumping of this large volume of blood imposes stresses and wear and tear on the various blood cells and on the endothelial cells of arteries. The relentless flow of blood through the vessels can damage platelets and endothelial cells and set the stage for the slow development of atheroma (lipid plaques).

This situation is aggravated in persons who have high levels of plasma LDL, high blood pressure, and platelets that are more sticky and aggregate. The development of atheroma and atherosclerosis represents a very complex process that proceeds over many years and involves the interplay of plasma lipoproteins, prostaglandins, white blood cells, platelets, and hemodynamic factors. Table 4.3 below shows the postulated mechanisms of atherosclerosis.

Table 4.3 Postulated mechanisms of atherosclerosis and CAD*

The intima is inflamed or damaged by chemical means or by turbulent blood flow

Platelets bind to and monocytes are attracted to the site of injury

Platelet binding leads to their producing thromboxane A_2

Thromboxane A2 stimulates platelet aggregation

Aggregated platelets release PDGF*and inflammatory cytokines

Aggregated platelets begin to form a thrombus plug

PDGF stimulates migration and proliferation of smooth medial muscle cells

Smooth muscle cells migrate to the intima and ingest oxidized LDL and VLDL

Monocytes and macrophages are attracted to the site of injury containing the aggregated platelets

Monocytes and macrophages become engorged with cholesterol from oxidized LDL and become foam cells that increase the growth of the plaque

Smooth muscle cells secrete collagen, elastin and proteoglycans, which enhance plaque growth

Plaques grow into complicated lesions containing lipids, dead cells, and calcium deposits

Plaque and thrombus growth narrows the lumen of the artery and eventually blocks the lumen which obstructs blood flow leading to a heart attack or stroke

* PDGF is platelet derived growth factor

*From Marinetti, G.V., 1990 Chapter 6, Table 6.5, page 131 with kind permission of Springer Science and Business Media.

Atherosclerosis has many aspects of an inflammatory disease (Paoletti et al 2004). Atherosclerosis is initiated by damage or inflammation of the intima of arteries and with elevated levels of white blood cells and aggregated platelets at the site of injury.

The inflammation mobilizes certain white blood cells (monocytes and macrophages) to the site of injury. Lipids accumulate in these cells and produce a yellow streak, the first sign of plaque formation. By age 10 most humans have some yellow lipid streaks in their arteries. Between ages of 10 and 25 the area of the intima covered by fatty streaks increases to about 10 to 50 percent. Some yellow streaks develop in the fibrous plaque, which is whitish in appearance and is elevated and consists of smooth muscle cells and foam cells. The cells are surrounded by collagen, elastic fibers, and proteoglycans. The matrix of these materials transforms the plaque into a fibrous cap, which can develop into the complicated lesion that has undergone calcification, hemorrhage, necrosis, and thrombosis. The plaque grows and blocks the blood flow in the artery causing a heart attack or stroke.

Damage to the intima, leading to development of an atheroma, has been called the response to injury hypothesis. Factors that can injury the endothelium of arteries have been shown to include hyperlipidemia (oxidized LDL), hypertension, smoking, chemical factors, immunologic factors, and infection. Severe high blood pressure may lead to high shear forces caused by vortex flow of blood. The high shear forces can damage the endothelial cells, platelets and red blood cells as they impinge on the endothelium.

Circulating immune complexes and antibodies can injure endothelial cells. Cigarette smoke may contain allergens that induce an immunoglobulin E response, which may injure endothelial cells.

Chemical injury to endothelial cells has been related to high levels of LDL and VLDL, and to chemicals such as homocystine, radiologic contrast dyes and chemotherapeutic drugs. Anoxia (oxygen depravation) can cause injury to endothelial cells. Carbon monoxide caused by cigarette smoking may lead to anoxia in arteries and damage the cells of the intima. Damage to the intima, leading to development of an atheroma, has been called the response to injury hypothesis.

Damage to endothelial cells can be produced by chemical agents such as homocystine and by physical agents such as a balloon catheter. These latter agents have been used experimentally in animals to induce atherosclerosis. The vitamin folic acid is believed to enhance the degradation of homocystine. Currently daily folic acid supplement (400 to 800 micrograms) is recommended to protect persons from getting atherosclerosis.

The involvement of platelets in atherogenesis is a crucial point of the thrombogenic hypothesis (Kher et al 2004). Platelet aggregation leads to the release of several factors that stimulate atherosclerosis. One factor is PDGF (platelet derived growth factor) that stimulates arterial smooth muscle cells to multiply and migrate to the site of injury on the intima, where they take up LDL particles and become foam cells. Smooth muscle cells also synthesize and secrete collagen, elastin, and proteoglycans, which form the matrix of the fibrous plaque.

The Oxidation of LDL May Initiate Plaque Formation

Oxidized LDL accumulate in arterial lesions and form at other inflammatory sites and initiate plaque formation in arteries. Whether the oxidized LDL is an initiator or accelerator of disease is the subject of speculation, debate, and intensive study. Oxidation may occur on the protein or on polyunsaturated fatty acids of phospholipids of LDL.

Studies have shown that high levels of plasma low density lipoprotein (LDL) correlates with the risk of atherosclerosis. The capacity of LDL to injure cells was directly related to the level of LDL oxidation. This led to the speculation for a possible role for oxidized LDL-mediated endothelial injury in atherogenesis.

Dr. Steinberg (1997) has been a leading scientist studying the oxidation of low density lipoproteins and the pathological significance of this oxidation. This research introduced the concept that oxidized LDL has altered composition and atherogenic properties.

The first demonstration that certain leukocyte populations could oxidize LDL used human neutrophils and activated populations of adherent human monocytes, cells well known to generate oxygen species. Chisolm et al (1999) take the position that monocytes-derived macrophages are likely candidates to mediate the in vivo oxidation of lipoproteins, because they are prominent in arterial lesions, known to generate activation-dependent reactive oxygen species. There may be multiple pathways through which monocytes-macrophages may promote extracellular LDL oxidation.

A consequence of an increase in the cholesterol ester content of macrophages is a dramatic increase in their synthesis and secretion of apoE. Takagi et al. (1988) have recently found that platelet-induced secretion of apoE paralleled the capacity of platelets to induce macrophage cholesterol accumulation. This finding provides new insight into the possible role of platelet-enhanced apoE production in atherosclerosis. However, which of the 6 types of apoE is involved needs to be studied.

The process of atherosclerosis is complex and is only partially understood. Many of the current concepts on the mechanisms of atherogenesis are provisional and undoubtedly will be modified in the near future.

Part 3

Biochemical Science Behind Heart Disease

Chapter 5

Metabolism of Fatty Acids

After foods are digested and absorbed into the blood they undergo a variety of metabolic reactions. Fatty acids are a major food in diet and provide more energy than do carbohydrates of proteins on a weight basis. An understanding of the metabolism of fatty acids is important to understanding the different types of diets and how they are related to weight gain and obesity. The types of fatty acids have been covered in the Introduction.

Most of the dietary fatty acids (FAs) have 16 to 24 carbon atoms and can be either saturated or unsaturated depending upon the presence of one or more double bonds in the fatty acid carbon chain.

The most abundant monounsaturated fatty acid is oleic acid. Oleic acid is the major fatty acid in olive oil. The two major classes of unsaturated fatty acids are n-3 and n-6. Linoleic acid and linolenic acid are called essential fatty acids since they cannot be made at all or in sufficient amount to sustain life by the human body and must be consumed in the diet.

Fatty acids are structural components of the more complex lipids including the phospholipids, triglycerides, diglycerides, monoglycerides, sphingolipids, and the glycosphingolipids. Fatty acids also are the precursors for the hormone-like eicosanoids, prostaglandins, leukotrienes, and lipoxins.

The n-3 and n-6 polyunsaturated fatty acids have biologically opposite properties, probably because they give rise to different eicosanoid products. When animals with a propensity to develop tumors are fed diets containing a large proportion of n-6 polyunsaturated fatty acids tumor formation is favored. However, when animals are fed diets with a similar proportion of n-3 polyunsaturated fatty acids tumor formation is inhibited.

Long-chain fatty acids are insoluble in water and are transported in plasma either esterified in triglycerides arranged in complex lipoproteins, or in a non-esterified form named NEFAs (non-esterified fatty acids) that are bound to albumin. Blood lipoproteins are synthesized from dietary lipids after absorption and esterification in the intestine or the liver. Saturated fatty acids can be made from excess glucose in the body.

General Aspects of Fatty Acid Metabolism

Excess dietary fatty acids and excess dietary carbohydrate are stored in adipose tissue as triglycerides. Insulin is the major hormone that stimulates this process of fat storage. Fatty acids are a prime fuel for humans and lower animals; they can be stored as triglycerides in large amounts in fat cells. The distribution of fuel storage in the body is shown in Table 5.1 below.

Table 5.1 Estimated fuel reserves in a 70 kg (154 lb) man in Calories*			
Tissue	**Protein**	**Glucose**	**Triglycerides**
Blood	0	60	45
Liver	400	400	450
Brain	0	8	0
Muscle	24,000	1200	450
Fat	40	80	135,000

*From Cahill, 1976. reproduced with permission, and from Marinetti, G.V. 1990 Chapter 2, Table 2-1, page 32 with kind permission of Springer Science and Business Media.

It is evident from the table that fats, as triglycerides, represent a much higher storage of energy than do carbohydrates and proteins. During starvation, glycogen and triglyceride stores are used first to supply the energy needs of the body. Glycogen reserves last only about 2 days whereas fat reserves can last for 1–2 months, depending on the body fat content. Proteins, especially the vital ones, are oxidized last, since their depletion is a threat to life.

However, some muscle proteins are oxidized during starvation. On the other hand muscle activity is greatly reduced under starvation conditions.

Some muscle proteins can be sacrificed to meet the energy demands of the brain and heart. It is also noteworthy that fats yield more energy and more water per gram when they are oxidized in the body than do the other foods as seen in Table 5.2 below.

Table 5.2 Energy and water produced when oxidized in the body*		
Food type	**Amount (kcal/gm)**	**Water/food (g/g)**
Carbohydrate	4.2	0.4
Proteins	4.3	0.4
Fat	9.2	1.1
Ethanol	7.0	0.9

* From Marinetti, G.V. 1990 Chapter 2, Table 2-2, page 32 with kind permission of Springer Science and Business Media.

The importance of fats as a prime storage form of energy is evident in nature. Migrating birds, hibernating animals, migrating seals, plant seeds, and eggs with a shell all contain high amounts of fats that serve the energy needs of the animal or cell. Migrating birds use this energy for muscle work. Eggs and seeds need this energy for growth of the embryo. A person lost in the woods without food or water can survive for one month or more without food but can survive for only about 7 to 10 days without water. Persons with more body fat can survive longer than those with less body fat. The oxidation of fat also produces more water than the oxidation of glucose. This is why camels can last a long time without food or water because they store a lot of fat in their humps.

When lower animals and humans require energy during stress or starvation, the stored fats in the body are mobilized by the action of certain hormones such as epinephrine (adrenalin). Binding of epinephrine induces a change in the membrane receptors that allows the receptors to activate the hormone sensitive lipase in the fat cells. The lipase hydrolyzes the triglycerides to diglycerides and free fatty acids. The fatty acids enter the blood and are taken up by various tissues for energy production. The body tissues that use fatty acids as a major source of energy are heart muscle, skeletal muscle, kidney, and liver. On the other hand brain uses mainly glucose for energy production.

Biological Oxidation of Fatty Acids

The metabolism of the fatty acids requires that they first be activated by conversion to coenzyme A esters. This reaction is catalyzed by enzymes. Oxidation of one mole of palmitic acid produces 774 kcal of energy as ATP. When one mole of palmitic acid is completely oxidized in a laboratory in a bomb calorimeter it releases 2348 kcal of energy. Therefore the biological oxidation of palmitic acid represents a 33 percent (774/2348) yield of chemical energy as ATP. Most of the other energy is converted to body heat.

Carnitine Cycle

L-carnitine (L stands for the levorotatory isomer) and acetyl carnitine and many other food supplements are sold in vitamin stores today. These stores provide little or no information on how these supplements work. Here I explain how carnitine functions in cells of the body.

Carnitine is a small organic compound that serves as the carrier of the fatty acids across the mitochondrial membrane. Mitochondria are small organelles in cells that are called the power houses of the cell because this is where foods are oxidized to produce energy and heat. The mitochondria contain enzymes that oxidize the end products of the breakdown of fatty acids and carbohydrates.

Fatty acid oxidation produces acetyl-CoA as the end product. Oxidation of carbohydrates produces glucose that first undergoes a series of enzyme reactions in the cytsol which produces pyruvic acid. This process is called glycolysis. Pyruvic acid enters the mitochondria and is converted to acetylCoA that is oxidized in another cycle of enzymes called the tricarboxylic acid cycle. The acetyl-CoA from fatty acids and from glucose is oxidized to carbon dioxide and water in the mitochondria. Dr. Bruce Ames and colleagues have shown that L-acetylcarnitine (or carnitine) protect mitochondria from oxidative damage. This topic is discussed more fully in Chapter 2.

The transport of fatty acids as fatty acid-CoA derivatives into the mitochondria requires two enzymes (called CAT-I and CAT-II) and a transport protein. Carnitine or acetyl-carnitine reacts with the fatty acid-CoA derivatives and form fatty acid-carnitine compounds that are able to interact with CAT-I and CAT-II and the transport protein that move the fatty acids into the mitochondria where they are reconverted to the fattyacidCoA derivatives and are oxidized inside the mitochondria. Some humans have been found to be deficient in carnitine and/or CAT-I. They develop muscle pain and weakness and accumulate fat in their muscles because the fatty acids cannot be properly oxidized. It is possible that diets lacking L-carnitine or aging can lead to carnitine deficiency and cause the muscle problems given above. If this occurs in the heart the symptoms could be more severe.

Biosynthesis of Fatty Acids

The body also makes fatty acids. The major fatty acid made from acetyl-CoA in the body is palmitic acid. The synthesis involves a reductive condensation process utilizing the coenzyme NADPH and is catalyzed by the fatty acid synthase multienzyme complex. The overall biosynthesis of palmitic acid is shown in Fig. 5.1 below.

Figure 5.1 Overall biosynthesis of palmitic acid

8Acetyl-CoA ———> Palmitic Acid + $7CO_2$ + 8CoA + $6H_2O$

Hormonal Regulation of Fatty Acid Synthesis and Oxidation

The human body can synthesize only certain types of fatty acids. The other fatty acids have to come from our diets. Fatty acids are synthesized from acetyl-CoA. The acetyl group is acetic acid that is found in vinegar. Acetyl groups can be produced from excess glucose or fat in the diet. The fatty acids are converted to triglycerides that are stored in fat cells. The liver, adipose tissue, and mammary glands are the major organs for this synthesis, and the hormone insulin plays an important role in stimulating the synthesis of fatty acids. Insulin also stimulates the synthesis of the enzymes that synthesize fatty acids and triglycerides.

The breakdown of triglycerides is stimulated by the hormones epinephrine (adrenalin) and glucagon during times of stress, exercise, and starvation.

Mobilization of Fatty Acids from Adipose Tissue

Mobilization of fatty acids from adipose tissue is regulated by hormones. Free fatty acids are released during fasting from the triglyceride stores it the fat cells. Fatty acid mobilization from fat cells also occurs during starvation and exercise.

The Functions of Polyunsaturated Fatty Acids

Dietary n-3 polyunsaturated fatty acids (n-3 PUFA) are polyunsaturated fatty acids containing 3 double bonds. They have an important impact on normal health and chronic disease. They regulate the levels of plasma lipids, immune function, insulin action, neuronal development, and visual function. Ingestion of n-3 PUFA will lead to their distribution to virtually every cell in the body with effects on membrane composition and function, eicosanoid synthesis, and in the regulation of gene expression. The n-3 fatty acids from fish protect humans from cancer, inflammation, blood clots, and heart disease.

Conversion of Fatty Acids to Eicosanoids

Eicosanoid is a collective term for fatty acid derivatives derived from certain polyunsaturated fatty acids such as arachidonic acid and linolenic acid. These derivatives are subdivided into prostaglandins, leukotrienes, lipoxins, and hydroxyl or peroxy derivatives of the fatty acids. The polyunsaturated fatty acids are substrates for the cyclooxygenase enzymes (labeled COX-1 and COX-2), and for the lipoxygenase enzymes. Cyclooxygenase products of the polyunsaturated fatty acids give rise to prostanoids called prostaglandins and thromboxanes.

Prostaglandins were first isolated from the prostate gland, thromboxanes were isolated form platelets (thrombocytes) and leukotrienes were isolated from white blood cells called leukocytes. The lipooxygenase (LOX) enzymes produce lipoxins and leukotrienes. The prostaglandins, lipoxins and leukotrienes are produced by most body organs in very small amounts and have hormone-like qualities.

Functions of Eicosanoids

The COX products are modulators of platelet aggregation, thrombosis, and chemotaxic responses, whereas the LOX products are involved in vascular permeability, vasoconstriction, inflammation, and bronchoconstriction. Eicosanoids produce a wide range of biological effects on inflammatory responses, on the intensity and duration of pain and fever, and on reproductive function (including the induction of labor). They also play important roles in inhibiting gastric acid secretion, regulating blood pressure and inhibiting or activating platelet aggregation and thrombosis. These enzymes are the targets for several anti-inflammatory drugs including Advil, Alleve, Viox, Celebrex and Bextra. Viox and Bextra have been discontinued because they caused deaths from heart disease in some patients. To date Celebrex appears to have fewer side effects than Viox or Bextra. Celebrex may need further investigation.

Essential Fatty Acid Deficiency

Two dietary polyunsaturated fatty acids, linoleic acid and linolenic acid, are essential for human life, since they cannot be synthesized by the body. Arachidonic acid, formed from linoleic acid, is not essential in humans if enough linoleic acid is taken in the diet. A deficiency of the essential fatty acids leads to skin lesions, fragile red blood cells, loss of hair, weight loss, kidney damage, sterility, and possibly death. The intake of 1–2 percent of the total dietary energy requirement as linoleic and linolenic acids is sufficient to prevent essential fatty acid deficiency. Linoleic acid and linolenic acid are essential in part because they are precursors for the eicosanoids. These essential fatty acids also help maintain a critical fluidity state in cell membranes.

Ketoacidosis

Under normal conditions, the oxidation of fatty acids in liver is regulated. However, when fatty acids go to the liver faster than the fatty acids can be oxidized a surplus of acetyl-CoA results. The excess acetyl-CoA is converted to organic acids called keto acids. The excessive production of ketoacids makes the blood acidic. This acidic blood condition is named ketoacidosis. **Ketoacidosis is a potentially life-threatening condition often causing afflicted persons to go into a coma. It is a serious problem in uncontrolled diabetes and in prolonged starvation.**

Fatty Acids and Tumor Formation

The two major classes of polyunsaturarted fatty acids (PUFAs) are n-3 and n-6. The n-3 and n-6 PUFAs have biologically opposite properties, probably because they give rise to different eicosanoid products. **As mentioned previously, when animals with a propensity to develop tumors are fed diets containing a large proportion of n-6 PUFAs, tumor formation is favored. However, when animals are fed diets with a similar proportion of n-3 polyunsaturated fatty acids, tumor formation is inhibited.**

Chapter 6

Cholesterol and Bile Acids

Overall Cholesterol Balance in Humans

The prime molecule involved in plaque formation in arteries during the process of atherosclerosis is cholesterol. Therefore I include a brief discussion of how cholesterol is handled in the body and how it is made and converted to lipoproteins. Also since cholesterol cannot be oxidized by the body as can fatty acids, it has to be converted to bile acids which are stored in the gall bladder.

Cholesterol is a white waxy sterol lipid that occurs in all animal cells but not in plants. It has an important structural role in cell membranes, is the precursor for steroid hormones in the adrenal gland, and is the precursor for bile acids in the liver. Because of its insolubility in water, it is solubilized and transported in the blood as a lipoprotein complex.

Cholesterol input to the body comes from the diet and from its synthesis, primarily by the liver. Cholesterol output occurs via secretion in the bile, conversion to bile acids, and loss from sloughing off of cells from the skin and intestines; a very small amount is lost in the urine. Lactating females also lose some cholesterol during breast feeding. The daily balance of cholesterol metabolism in humans is shown below in Table 6.1.

Table 6.1 Daily balance of cholesterol metabolism*	
DIET **500–1000 mg**	**METABOLISM TO** **Bile acids 600 mg** **Steroids hormones 40 mg**
Synthesis by the liver **1000 mg**	**Excretion** **Fecal sterols 500 mg** **Skin 80 mg/** **Urine1 mg** **Milk 80 mg**

* From Marinetti, 1990, Chapter 4, Figure 4-1, page 64 with kind permission of springer Scence and Business Media.

A 70-kg adult human contains about 140 g of total cholesterol, of which about 8 g is present in plasma. The average daily diet contains about 500 to 1000 mg of cholesterol and the liver synthesizes about 1000 mg/day. Since the daily metabolic need for cholesterol is approximately 350 mg, the balance has to be excreted, mainly via the bile. The recommended daily requirement for cholesterol is set at no more than 300 mg/day. This is not a well established number since it depends on the type of food taken and on the size of the person.

Biosynthesis of Cholesterol

The synthesis of cholesterol occurs in the liver. It is estimated that the synthesis requires about 26 separate reactions. Some of the steps in the synthesis of cholesterol are depicted in below in Fig. 6.1. These are shown so that the reader can appreciate the complexity of how cholesterol is made in the body.

Figure 6.1 Overall biosynthesis of cholesterol*

2 Acetyl-CoA (C-2)————> Acetoacetyl-CoA (C-4)

Acetyl-CoA + Acetoacetyl-CoA ————> HMG-CoA (C-6)

HMG-CoA + 2NADPH ————> Mevalonic acid (C-6)

Mevalonic acid + ATP ————> Mevalonatephosphate

Mevalonatephosphate + ATP ————> Mevalonatepyrophosphate

Mevalonatepyrophosphate ————> Isopentenylpyrophosphate (C-5)

2 Isopentenypyrophosphate ————> Geranylpyrophosphate (C-10)

Geranylpyrophosphate + C-5 ————> Farnesylpyrophosphate (C-15)

2 Farnesylpyrophosphate ————> Squalene(C-30)

Squalene ————> Lanosterol (C-30)

Lanosterol ————> Cholesterol (C-27)

***C-2 signifies two carbon atoms etc. for the others**

* From Marinetti, 1990 Chapter 4, Figure 4-3, page 65 with kind permission of Springer Science and Business Media.

The water-soluble products are made in the cytosol, whereas the lipid-soluble products are made in the endoplasmic reticulum membrane. Phosphorylated intermediates play an important role in the early part of synthesis up to the formation of farnesyl pyrophosphate. As the intermediates in the synthesis become more hydrophobic the process occurs in the endoplasmic reticulum.

The rate-limiting regulatory step in the synthesis of cholesterol is the conversion of HMG-CoA (hydroxymethylglutaryl coenzyme CoA) to mevalonic acid. Statin drugs used to lower blood cholesterol, inhibit this reaction. The rate limiting reaction determines how fast and how much cholesterol is made by the body. It is the important rate-limiting reaction that regulates the enzyme. Statin drugs inhibit this enzyme. The reaction is shown below in Fig. 6.2.

Figure 6.2 Rate-limiting reaction in the biosynthesis of cholesterol*

HMG-CoA + 2NADPH ————> Mevalonic acid + 2 NADP$^+$ + 2H$^+$

*From Marinetti, 1990 Chapter 4, Figure 4-4, page 65 with kind permission of Springer Science and Business Media.

The enzyme catalyzing this reaction is HMG-CoA reductase (HMGR). Insulin stimulates the synthesis of HMGR. Through a series of complex steps, lanosterol (C-30) is ultimately converted to cholesterol which has twenty seven carbon atoms (C-27).

Cholesterol and triglycerides are very insoluble in water. For this reason, their synthesis occurs with enzymes localized on cell membranes and is synchronized with the synthesis of phospholipids and specific proteins and are assembled into chylomicrons in the intestine and are made into VLDL and HDL lipoproteins in the liver. The lipoproteins are then secreted into the bloodstream where they carry cholesterol and phospholipids to other cells of the body. Cholesterol also is used for the synthesis of steroid hormones in the adrenal gland, testes, and ovaries.

Regulation of Cholesterol Biosynthesis by Sterol Regulatory Elements SREs)

Sterol regulatory elements (SREs) in DNA regulate the transcription (DNA making mRNA) of mRNAs for LDL receptors, for HMGCoA reductase. and other enzymes of cholesterol synthesis. SREs are specific DNA segments in promoter regions of target genes. SREBPs (sterol response element binding proteins) are specific proteins that bind to SREs. See the Introduction for more information relating to DNA, RNA, and transcription.

SREBPs bind to promoter regions on DNA for the synthesis of LDL receptors and for the enzymes that make cholesterol. The LDL receptors are special proteins on cell membranes which bind LDL and allow it to enter the cell where it is metabolized.

Bile and Bile Acids

Bile is a green-yellow viscous secretion of the liver. Human bile contains about 100 ml of fluid, bile acids, cholesterol, phospholipids, and the bile pigments bilirubin and biliverdin. Liver produces 0.4 to 1 gm of bile salts per day and secretes about 15 to 30 grams per day into the intestines. Fortunately most of the secreted bile acids are reabsorbed from the intestines into the blood. The bile acids emulsify the fats in the diet.

Intestinal bacteria also convert an appreciable amount of cholesterol (dietary or from bile) into two other sterols, cholestanol and coprostanol. These sterols are poorly absorbed and are lost in the feces and thus tend to lower cholesterol levels in the blood. In the adrenal gland, cholesterol serves as the substrate for the synthesis of adrenal steroid hormones. Ultraviolet light converts choles-terol to vitamin D in the skin.

Chapter 7

Blood Lipoproteins:
and High levels of Blood Lipids

Types of Blood Lipoproteins

The insolubility of cholesterol in water is overcome by the body combining cholesterol with phospholipids and proteins to make lipoproteins which are more soluble and that are metabolized by enzymes. Because of the importance of the blood lipoproteins called LDL and HDL in the development of athero-sclerosis and heart disease, it is helpful to know something of the properties and metabolism of these lipoproteins.

Blood lipoproteins represent a variety of large heterogeneous molecules that have the major function of transporting the water-insoluble lipids (particularly triglycerides, cholesterol, and cholesterol esters) in the blood. Lipoproteins are dynamic molecules in a constant state of synthesis and degradation actively exchanging certain lipids and proteins with each other. On the basis of density they are named chylomicrons, very low density lipoproteins (VLDL) inter-mediate density lipoproteins (IDL) and high density lipoproteins (HDL). The protein and total lipid content of the blood lipoproteins are listed in Table 7.1 below.

Table 7.1 Protein and lipid content of blood lipoproteins		
Lipoprotein	**Percent Protein**	**Percent Total Lipid**
Chylomicrons	1–2	98–99
VLDL	7–10	90–93
IDL	11	89
LDL	21	79
HDL	33–75	43–67

*In part from Murray et al 1988 reproduced with permission and from Marinetti, G.V. Chapter 5, Table 5-1, page 77 with with kind permission from Springer Science and Business Media.

The lipoproteins are separated on the basis of their densities. On the basis of density they are named chylomicrons, very-low-density lipoproteins (VLDL), intermediate-density lipoproteins (IDL), and high-density lipoproteins (HDL). The characteristics of the lipoproteins are listed in the Table 7.1 above.

Chylomicrons and VLDL are high in lipid and low in protein. Lipoproteins are major carriers of triglycerides and cholesterol in the blood. Chylomicrons carry triglycerides from the intestines to the liver, whereas VLDL transport triglycerides and some cholesterol from the liver to other tissues of the body. LDL are small particles that are high in cholesterol and cholesterol esters; they are the principal carriers of cholesterol in the blood. Most lipoproteins have a higher content of cholesterol esters (cholesterol containing a long chain fatty acid as an ester bond).

HDL are the smallest particles and contain the highest content of protein. Chylomicrons are the largest and lightest particles and give the plasma a milky appearance. VLDL and IDL, because of their intermediate size and density, give the plasma a turbid appearance. LDL and HDL, even when present in abnormally high levels do not confer turbidity to the plasma. **High levels of LDL are associated with premature atherosclerosis and coronary artery disease (CAD) whereas high levels of HDL provide protection from these diseases.**

Enzymes that breakdown blood lipoproteins: Lipases LPL and HL

Lipoprotein lipase (LPL) occurs in the blood and hydrolyzes the triglycerides on blood lipoproteins (mainly chylomicrons and VLDL). Insulin stimulates the release of LPL into the blood where in the presence of apoC-II it hydrolyzes the triglycerides on lipoproteins to produce free fatty acids and glycerol. The gene for LPL occurs on chromosome 8 in humans. Genetic defects in LPL lead to very high levels of triglycerides in the blood.

Liver hepatic lipase (HL) degrades blood chylomicron remnants that are taken up by liver cells. Rare genetic deficiencies of HL are characterized by abnormal levels of LDL, HDL and VLDL.

Metabolism of Chylomicrons

The dietary triglyceride-rich lipoproteins, called chylomicrons, are the largest lipoproteins (>100 nm in diameter). They are synthesized in the small intestine and carry primarily triglycerides and cholesterol via the lymphatics to the blood. Chylomicrons are degraded in the blood by the enzyme LPL, which hydrolyzes the triglycerides to free fatty acids and glycerol and converts the chylomicrons to smaller particles called chylomicron remnants.

The fatty acids that are released can be taken up by many cells, but adipocytes (fat cells) take up the most of the fatty acids and store them as triglycerides. The chylomicron remnants are taken up by liver cells that have specific membrane receptors. The chylomicron remnants are taken up by a process called receptor-mediated endocytosis. ApoC-II activates lipoprotein lipase.

Elevated levels of chylomicrons give blood plasma a milky appearance and cause hypertriglyceridemia, since these lipoproteins are very high in triglycerides. Genetic defects in the synthesis of LPL give rise to a severe hypertriglyceridemia called hyperlipoproteinemia type Ia. A deficiency of apoC-II gives rise to hyperlipoproteinemia type Ib, in which plasma levels of triglycerides (as chylomicrons) are greatly elevated.

Metabolism of Very Low-Density Lipoproteins (VLDL)

The endogenous lipoproteins named VLDL are produced in the liver. They transport triglycerides, phospholipids, and cholesterol from the liver to other tissues of the body. VLDL are degraded by LPL stepwise, first into IDL (intermediate density lipoproteins) and then to LDL (low density lipoproteins). The conversion of VLDL to LDL is shown below in Fig. 7.1.

Figure 7.1 Metabolism of VLDL

VLDL ———> IDL ———> LDL

The proteins of VLDL are synthesized in the liver. The lipids and apoproteins are assembled, packaged, and transported to the plasma membrane and released into the blood.

The VLDL and IDL particles in type III disease are abnormal and have been called β-VLDL. Apparently, these particles are avidly taken up by macrophages and produce foam cells that are laden with cholesterol and cholesterol esters and stimulate the process of atherosclerosis.

Metabolism of "Good" HDL (High-Density Lipoproteins)

HDL represent several lipoprotein species that differ in their protein and lipid content, shape, structure, and density. They are made in the liver and, to some extent, in the small intestine.

HDL and Reverse Cholesterol Transport

When HDL transfer cholesterol esters to VLDL and LDL, the HDL lose cholesterol and thus are able to pick up additional cholesterol from peripheral tissues and transport them to liver, where the cholesterol can be converted to bile acids. **This process, called reverse cholesterol transport, is believed to explain why high levels of HDL offer protection from coronary heart disease and is called the "good cholesterol".**

The transport of cholesterol from peripheral tissues to the liver is the major way for the body to eliminate excess cholesterol, since only the liver can convert cholesterol to bile acids. Some LDL are also taken up by a non-receptor-mediated pathway (called by some the scavenger pathway) in arterial endothelial cells and liver cells.

Metabolism of "Bad" LDL (Low-Density Lipoproteins)

Animal cells have specific mechanisms for obtaining the cholesterol required for synthesis of cell membranes, steroid hormones, and bile acids. Cells can synthesis cholesterol or they can take up dietary cholesterol from the blood by receptor-mediated endocytosis. LDL must first bind to a specific receptor, the LDL receptor on the cell plasma membrane. There are approximately 40,000 receptors per cell.

Either the free cholesterol is incorporated into the various cell membranes or the excess is transported out of the cell to the liver by HDL-mediated reverse cholesterol transport. Most cells use the cholesterol made in the liver.

The regulation of receptor synthesis allows the cells to take up only the amount of cholesterol needed. In normal cells, the LDL receptor and HMGR are under feedback regulation so that when cholesterol levels in the cell rise too high, syntheses of the LDL receptor and HMGR are repressed. **If this balance is not maintained, hypercholesterolemia (high level of blood cholesterol) will occur. The cholesterol in LDL is named the "bad cholesterol" because elevated levels of LDL-cholesterol are associated with high risk for atherosclerosis, heart disease and stroke.**

Hyperlipoproteinemias (High Levels of Blood Lipoproteins)

Hyperlipoproteinemia represents the abnormal elevation of one or more of the blood lipoproteins that transport cholesterol and triglycerides in the blood. Beaumont, Fredrickson and co-workers (1970) have arbitrarily classified the hyperlipoproteinemias into five types labeled as I–V (or 1–5). The primary causes of elevated blood lipids include genetic defects, eating foods that contain too much saturated and trans fatty acids, eating too much refined carbohydrates (potato, pasta, and white rice) and lack of exercise. The secondary causes of elevated cholesterol and or triglycerides are shown in Table 7.2 below.

Table 7.2 Secondary causes of elevated blood lipids
Obesity
Diabetes or insulin resistance
Hypothyroidism
Kidney disease, nephritic syndrome
Excess alcohol intake
Excess beta-adrenergic antagonists drugs
Thiazide diuretics
Steroid medications, corticosterids
Zoloft therapy
Cigarette smoking

Obesity, diabetes, excess alcohol intake, and smoking are the more prevalent secondary causes of elevated blood lipids. Ii is noteworthy that drugs other than lipid lowering drugs can influence blood lipid levels.

The cutoff values for defining overt hyperlipidemia can vary in different clinical laboratories and are only approximate guides for physicians. **It is now generally accepted that a cholesterol value of over 240 mg/dl for any age group is above normal. The total cholesterol level should be below 200 mg/dl. Indeed, some researchers now believe that this level should be below 170 mg/dl.**

This recommendation has implications on drug therapy for hypercholesterolemia since to reduce the level of total cholesterol to the 150–170 mg/dl range would force patients to take higher doses of drugs like the Statins. This increases the cost and also the risk of having more side effects.

The deleterious effects of the hyperlipoproteinemias develop slowly, often requiring many years. The major problem is atherosclerosis, which leads to coronary artery disease and strokes. Several epidemiological studies suggest that the risk of coronary heart disease begins to increase sharply at cholesterol levels above 200 mg/dl. Thus, hypercholesterolemia may be defined as any level over 200 mg/dl.

An LDL/HDL cholesterol ratio of greater than 3 increases the risk of heart disease. The risk for coronary heart disease increases markedly as the LDL/HDL cholesterol ratio rises above 5.

A link between plasma triglyceride level and atherosclerosis is now well established. It appears that hypertriglyceridemia is present in a disproportionate number of patients with coronary heart disease. This finding may be attributable in part to the particular lipoprotein species found to be elevated that carries the triglyceride.

Hyperlipoproteinemias (high levels of blood lipoproteins)

Cholesterol and triglycerides are carried by lipoproteins in the blood because cholesterol and triglycerides are not soluble in water. This is why blood analysis refers to LDL cholesterol, VLDL cholesterol, or HDL cholesterol. High levels of blood cholesterol or triglycerides cause the hyperlipoproteinemias.

Bad eating habits, genetic makeup, age, sex, lack of physical activity, and hormonal imbalance contribute to hyperlipoproteinemia. Some of these factors are interrelated. Epidemiological studies have favored the dietary causation of hyperlipidemia, while clinical investigators and basic scientists have emphasized the genetic and biochemical factors. Dietary factors should not be dissociated from the genetic factors.

It is evident that if one overeats, the excess intake of food puts a strain on the metabolic system of the body even if no genetic abnormality is present and that the strain is much greater if a genetic defect is present. Moreover, the types and amount of dietary food including saturated fats, trans fatty acids, and the specific types of polyunsaturarted fatty acids (n-3 versus n-6), cholesterol, and daily exercise have a profound influence on the metabolic systems that handle the ingested food.

High levels of blood triglycerides can be treated by restricting dietary fats and replacing the ordinary dietary fats with medium-chain triglycerides (MCT). These triglycerides have fatty acids with chain length of 12 carbon atoms or less. When the medium-chain triglycerides are hydrolyzed in the intestines, the fatty acids are absorbed directly into the blood and hence bypass the chylomicron formation. These persons must be supplied with sufficient essential fatty acids (linoleic and linoleic acids).

Genetic defects of LDL and the LDL receptor

Genetic defects are known to occur in both apoB of LDL or in the membrane receptor for apoB. This receptor has been named the LDL receptor. When the LDL receptor binds the ApoB protein on LDL it allows the LDL to get into the cell where LDL is metabolized.

The LDL receptor in humans has been shown to have several genetic mutations. Nine mutations have been identified by molecular cloning and DNA sequence analysis. The early research of Goldstein and Brown (1983, 1984; Brown and Goldstein, 1984, 1986, 1987) has elucidated the genetic defect in LDL. They received the Nobel Prize for this research in 1985.

Persons with genetic defects of LDL or the LDL receptor have type IIa hyperlipoproteinemia evidenced by very high levels of both plasma LDL cholesterol and plasma total cholesterol Plasma is the supernatant fluid that is formed when blood is centrifuged at high speed. Spinning the blood forms three distinct layers; a top clear or cloudy layer, a thin middle layer of white blood cells, and a lower layer of red blood cells. The top layer is called plasma and contains the lipoproteins. When I mention blood lipids this means plasma lipids. I use the term blood since most persons may be more familiar with the term blood than with the term plasma.

Homozygous (genes from both parents are defective) individuals have cholesterol levels in the range of 800–1200 mg/dl and suffer from early onset of atherosclerosis and coronary heart disease. Xanthomas (cholesterol and other lipid deposits) appear on the skin within the first 4 years of life, and coronary heart disease can occur at this early age.

Patients who are heterozygous have only one defective gene and hence have half the number of LDL receptors. These patients have cholesterol levels of 400–600 mg/dl. Many develop atherosclerosis and coronary heart disease later in life, usually in their 50s or 60s but can develop tendinous xanthomas in their 30s.

Type IIb hyperlipoproteinemia is associated with increased levels of both plasma cholesterol and triglycerides resulting from increased levels of LDL and either IDL or VLDL. This lipid disorder, also called combined hyperlipidemia, is seen in early development of atherosclerosis and coronary heart disease.

The uptake of apoE and chylomicron remnants by liver cells is important in regulating the levels of cholesterol and triglycerides in the blood. There are three major isoforms of apoE (E2, E3, and E4). The E2 and E4 types are associated with hypertriglyceridemia and hypercholesterolemia, respectively. ApoE4 is believed to be involved in type V hyperlipoproteinemia (Kuusi et al., 1988).

Chapter 8

Excess Carbohydrate is Converted to Fat and Causes Obesity

This last chapter is included because obesity is a major cause of heart disease and diabetes in the U.S. Also excess carbohydrate in the diet is converted to fat and this leads to overweight and obesity. Understanding the science behind this process is necessary to convince the public to watch how much and what type of carbohydrate they consume in their diets.

The Glycemic Index

Carbohydrates are classified by their glycemic index. This index is based on the response that the ingested carbohydrate produces on the levels of blood sugar (glucose) and insulin. Carbohydrates having a high glycemic index produce a higher level of blood glucose and insulin than those with a low glycemic index.

Complex polymer type carbohydrates have a lower glycemic index than simple sugars like table sugar (sucrose) or glucose. Some refined carbohydrates such as those found in pasta, rice, and potato have a higher glycemic index than carbohydrates found in vegetables and beans. Carbohydrates with a high glycemic index are more likely to lead to overweight and obesity and increase the risk of developing diabetes.

How excess dietary carbohydrate (glucose) is converted to fat.

The metabolism of fatty acids and glucose are interrelated. Excess glucose in the body is converted to fatty acids and stored as triglycerides in fat cells called adipocytes. The main fatty acid produced from glucose is palmitic acid, a saturated fatty acid. The palmitic acid along with other fatty acids are converted to and stored as triglycerides in fat cells. This process can lead to excessive weight gain (obesity) because fat cells can proliferate (make new cells) and store a lot of fat. Obesity increased in the U.S. when many persons followed the low fat diets in the 1980s and increased their consumption of refined carbohydrates to get more calories. Unfortunately this led to the metabolic syndrome and to type-2 diabetes in both children and adults. See chapter 2 for more information on the metabolic syndrome.

Glucose and fatty acid metabolism are interrelated and are regulated by the hormones insulin, epinephrine (adrenalin), glucagons, and by transcription factors. Insulin and glucagon are made in the pancreas and have opposing effects on metabolism of lipids and glucose. Insulin is released into the blood when the glucose level rises after eating a carbohydrate meal. The elevated blood glucose level triggers the pancreas to produce and release insulin. Insulin converts the glucose to glycogen in the liver and the blood level of glucose decreases to normal.

Glucagon is released during starvation and stimulates the breakdown of glycogen to produce glucose. This raises the level of blood glucose. Insulin levels increase after a meal whereas glucagon and epinephrine levels decrease after a meal. Moreover, glucagon and epinephrine inhibit the release of insulin from the pancreas.

Insulin must get out of the pancreas and into the blood to carry out its functions. In type 2 diabetes the release of insulin from the islet cells in the pancreas is decreased or possibly the released insulin does not react with its target fat cells in a normal way. Either the insulin transport protein is defective or the body produces antibodies to the insulin transport protein or to insulin. This is an autoimmune disease.

Insulin increases the levels of the enzymes that make triglycerides by fat cells. The fat cells rely on the liver to make the fatty acids and glycerol, which are needed to make triglycerides. Insulin also activates the enzymes which make triglycerides in the fat cells.

The human body cycles between feeding and starvation stages. During feeding the genes for the storage of dietary glucose as glycogen and the storage of fatty acids as triglycerides are activated by transcription factors that stimulate the genes to make the enzymes required for these processes. During starvation the reverse occurs and the genes for synthesis and storage of foods are depressed and the breakdown and oxidation of foods are stimulated.

The transcription factors for the breakdown and oxidation of foods activate the genes for the enzymes of these metabolic processes. Transcription factors can be large protein molecules or small organic molecules. Fatty acids and glucose are now known to regulate the synthesis or activation of transcription factors.

Glucose is oxidized to provide energy for brain, skeletal muscle and heart muscle and indeed for all the organs of the body. The oxidation of glucose provides chemical energy in the form of ATP. The complete oxidation of one mole of fatty acid produces about 10 times the amount of chemical energy as ATP compared to the oxidation of one mole of glucose.

During starvation glycogen breakdown provides glucose for the energy needed for the body. Glucose undergoes a process called glycolysis. This occurs in the cytosol of cells and produces pyruvic acid. Pyruvic acid enters the mitochondria where it is converted to acetyl-CoA that is oxidized completely in the mitochondria of cells to produce energy.

When excess acetyl-CoA is produced from glucose it is converted to fatty acids. The fatty acids are converted to triglycerides and stored in fat cells. Fat cells can store a very large amount of fat because the body can produce more fat cells. However, the liver and muscles can store a very limited amount of glycogen. In a 72 kg man, fat cells can store 135,000 kcal of energy compared to only 450 kcal from muscle. See Chapter 5, table 5.2.

Glucose, fatty acids, and cholesterol play a role in regulating the transcription of genes involved in their metabolism. Glucose regulates the transcription of a number of genes that are controlled by insulin. Several transcription factors have been proposed as intermediates in the control of the expression of genes by glucose. The sterol regulatory element binding protein (SREBP) is a transcription factor for both glucose and insulin action on specific genes in the liver and adipose tissue.

Regulation of the metabolism of cholesterol, glucose, and fatty acids

SREs and SREBPs are involved in the regulation of the metabolism of the cholesterol, glucose and fatty acids. The term SRE meant sterol regulatory element because it was first found to regulate the metabolism of cholesterol. Later SREs were found to regulate the metabolism of glucose and fatty acids. A more inclusive term for SRE should be substrate regulating element and a more inclusive term for SREBP should be substrate regulatory element binging protein.

SREs are specific DNA segments in promoter regions of target genes that regulate the transcription (DNA making mRNA) of mRNAs for glucose, fatty acid and cholesterol metabolism. SREBPs are specific proteins that bind to

SREs and activate these genes. Future studies will undoubtedly find new SREs and SREBPS for other important substrates involved in the metabolism of proteins and nucleic acids.

Insulin-and glucose transport proteins (GLUTs)

Insulin regulates the overall metabolism of glucose. This is achieved by stimulation of specific proteins called glucose transport proteins (GLUTs). These transport proteins regulate glucose uptake into cells from a variety of organs the main ones being muscle, brain, red blood cells, and fat cells. In mammalian systems there are currently about nine distinct glucose transport proteins.

Insulin stimulates glucose transport into these cells by causing the migration of GLUT4 from an intracellular compartment to the plasma membrane. The transport proteins get inserted into the plasma membrane, where they bind glucose and facilitate the uptake of glucose into the cells. This process is necessary for the utilization of blood glucose and for controlling the level of blood glucose.

Insulin also stimulates the migration of GLUT4s from the cell membrane to the cytosol. Patients with type 2 diabetes have decreased insulin-stimulated glucose transport. This is a major metabolic defect may be caused by long term eating of excess carbohydrates.

In the pancreatic beta cells, glucose is the primary physiological stimulus for the regulation of insulin synthesis and secretion. In the liver, glucose induces expression of genes that code for glucose transport proteins and for the enzymes that metabolize glucose. The glucose transport proteins of brain and red blood cells bind glucose more tightly than other transport proteins. This insures that brain and red blood cells receive the glucose they need to survive. Brain and red blood cells oxidize glucose whereas skeletal muscle, heart muscle, liver, and fat cells oxidize both fatty acids and glucose.

Insulin represses the genes of the gluconeogenic and fatty acid pathways. The gluconeogenic pathway produces glucose from the breakdown products of certain amino acids and from glycerol from the metabolism of fat. Gluconeogenesis is important in maintaining normal glucose levels during starvation. In the fed state, gluconeogenesis would produce too much glucose that may increase the risk of type-2 diabetes. Insulin prevents this by inhibiting gluconeogenesis.

Epilogue

My life experience with heart disease and my profession as a biochemist prompted me to write this book. It is my hope that my book will help others understand the health risks of high levels of blood cholesterol and triglycerides and take advantage of the benefits of diets, drugs, and exercise that help prevent heart disease. I was able to beat heart disease and so can you.

Afterword

Each person must take responsibility to care for his or her health. A strong commitment to staying with diet therapy, doing exercises, and getting medical help without delay are all essential for a successful treatment and prolonging life. This commitment requires a lot of will power and staying informed on the new scientific developments on new diets and new drugs.

Conclusion

In today's world of rapid growing technology and medical advances the lay public needs to have a basic elementary knowledge of science. I have included the more practical and vital information on heart disease in chapters 2 and 3 of my book and purposely have put the biochemical background in part 3 of my book. I believe that the lay public should understand how foods are metabolized by the human body. I also believe that this knowledge will empower people how best to use and understand the diets and the drugs that are used today to treat heart disease.

The public today hears terms like HDL cholesterol, LDL cholesterol, omega-3 fatty acids, obesity, glycemic index, and the metabolic syndrome, but do they really know what these mean?

The lay public may find parts 1 and 2 of this book more to their interest than part 3. However, I encourage all readers to look at all three parts of this book so that they can better understand the scientific basis of diets and drugs used to treat high levels of blood lipids and heart disease. To help the readers I have included in the Introduction of the book a section on some basic concepts of biochemistry and the types of lipids.

Glossary

Acetyl-CoA, the end product of the metabolism of glucose and fatty acids and the substrate for the synthesis of fatty acids and cholesterol

Adenine, nitrogen containing organic cyclic compound that occurs in DNA and RNA

Adipose tissue, fat tissue which stores excess fat in the body

Adiposite, a fat cell

Anabolism, the synthetic chemical reactions in cells that make all the chemicals in cells

Anemia, a low level of red cells in the blood

Bile acids, products formed from cholesterol in the liver and that emulsify dietary fats for digestion

Biosynthesis, the synthesis of molecules by living cells, utilizing enzymes and substrates

Carbohydrates, polymers of glucose including starches, glycogen, and dextrins

Catabolism, the degradative chemical reactions in cells which breakdown compounds

Cell membrane, a thin bimolecular layer of phospholipids and cholesterol that surrounds all cells and contains proteins and glycoproteins

Cholesterol, a lipid consisting of a large heterocyclic ring and is carried by lipoproteins in the blood. It is converted to bile acids and in the skin is converted to vitamin D by sunlight

Coronary arteries, arteries that branch off the aorta and supply blood to the heart muscles

Deoxyribonucleic acid, the genetic material of all cells

Docosahexenoic acid (DHA), a fatty acid having twenty two carbon atoms and six double bonds and occurs mainly in fish fat

Double bond, a chemical bond formed by two atoms sharing a pair of electrons

Eicosanoids, a family of products derived from polyunsaturated fatty acids, which consist of prostaglandins, leukotrienes, and lipoxins and have many biological functions

Eicosapentenoic acid (EPA) a fatty acid containing twenty carbon atoms and five double bonds and is found mainly in fish oil

Endoplasmic reticulum, a layer of membranes found in all cells where lipids and proteins are made, the latter with the aid of ribosomes

Enzyme, a protein with catalytic activity which acts specifically on a compound called the substrate; enzymes lower the energy of activation of the chemical reaction that allows the reaction to occur at a rapid rate at body temperature

Epinephrine a hormone made in the adrenal gland and also called adrenalin

Fatty acid, a lipid made from four to 24 carbon atoms arranged in a linear fashion and having no double bond or having up to six double bonds. Most fatty acids in humans contain an even number of carbon atoms.

Fibrinogen, a protein in the blood which is converted to fibrin by the enzyme thrombin during the formation of a blood clot

Gastric, referring to the stomach

Gene, a specific arrangement of a triad of nucleotides in DNA that codes for a specific protein

Ghrelin, a protein hormone involved in the metabolism of fat

Glands, organs in the body that make hormones

Glucagon, a hormone made in the pancreas which regulates blood glucose

Glycemic index, the level of blood glucose and insulin produced by a given amount of a carbohydrate in the diet

Glycolysis, the breakdown of glucose to pyruvic acid in the cytosol of cells

Golgi, a stack of membranes in the cell that regulates the processing of proteins

Good carbohydrates, contain a low glycemic index and are high in fiber and unrefined starch

Good fats, contain omega-3 fatty acids especially the EPA and DHA found in fish oil, and do not contain trans fatty acids and have very small amount of saturated fatty acids

Good proteins contain all the essential amino acids and are found in fish and poultry

Gram, a unit of weight equal to 0.0022 lbs.; 1 kilogram equals 2.2 lbs.

Guanine, nitrogen containing cyclic organic compound found in DNA and RNA

Hemostasis, the regulation of the coagulation of the blood

Hepatic, refers to liver

Hormone, a molecule produced in very small amounts by glands of the body

Hypercholesterolemia, high blood levels of cholesterol

Hyperglycemia, high levels of blood glucose (sugar)

Hyperlipidemia, high levels of blood lipids (cholesterol and trglycerides)

Hypertriglyceridemia, high levels of blood triglycerides

Hypoglycemia, low levels of blood glucose

Hypothalamus, a region of the brain

Ileum, part of the small intestine

Insulin, a hormone produced by the pancreas that regulates glucose and lipid metabolism

Jejunum, part of the small intestine

Ketoacidosis, the increase in acidity of the blood resulting from excess ketoacids

Ketosis, accumulation of ketoacids in the blood

Kilogram, 1000 grams that is equal to 2.2 lbs.

Leptin, a hormone which regulates the metabolism of fat and satiety (feeling full after eating)

Leukotrienes, products of polyunsaturated fatty acids which have hormone-like properties

Lipid bilayers, A molecular stacking of two phospholipid molecules that occur in membranes

Lipoproteins, large molecular aggregates containing lipids and proteins that transport lipids in the blood

Lipoxins, hormone-like molecules produced from polyunsaturated fatty acids

Membrane bilayers, pairs of phospholipids stacked tail to tail making a lipid bilayer

Metabolic syndrome, a metabolic condition characterized by overweight, high level of blood glucose and blood lipids, low level of HDL,

Metabolism, the sum of all chemical reactions of the body

Milligram, one thousandth of a gram

Mitochondria, power house organelles in cells that oxidize foods and produce energy

Molarity, refers to the concentration of chemical solutions.

n-3 Fatty acids. fatty acids in which the last double bond is three carbon atoms from the terminal carbon atom of the fatty acid chain

n-6 Fatty acids, fatty acids in which the last double bond is six carbon atoms from the terminal carbon atom of the fatty acid chain

Nanomolar, one millionth of molarity, or 10^{-6} molar.

Peroxisomes, organelles in cells which can oxidize fatty acids and which contain the enzyme catalase which degrades hydrogen peroxide

Phospholipid, a lipid containing glycerol, fatty acids, phosphate and nitrogen base such as choline, serine, ethanolamine, or inositol

Picomolar, one billionth of molarity or 10^{-12} molar

Pituitary gland, the master gland of the brain

Plasma, the supernatant fluid obtained when whole blood is centrifuged

Plasmin, an enzyme which hydrolyzes blood clots

Platelet plug. A clot formed by aggregated platelets

Platelets, small non-nucleated cell-like structures in blood that are important if forming clots from injuries.

Polyunsaturated fatty acids, fatty acids containing two or more double bonds

Prostacyclin, a prostaglandin which stimulates platelet aggregation

Prostaglandins, hormone-like compounds produced from certain polyunsaturated fatty acids

Protein receptors, proteins occurring on cell membranes which bind hormones that leads to the activation of one or more enzymes

Protein, a large molecule containing a linear sequence of many amino acids

Prothrombin, the inactive form of thrombin

Rate limiting reaction, the reaction in a series of reactions that regulates how fast the process will occur

Replication, the ability of DNA to make more of its own structure

Ribonucleic acid (RNA) nucleic acid polymers made of the sugar ribose, the bases adenine, guanine, uracil, and cytosine which are linked by a diphosphate bond. There are several types of RNA. One called mRNA has the genetic information to make proteins.

Ribosomes, small complex structures in cells that interact with mRNA to make proteins

Serum, the supernatant fluid obtained when clotted blood is centrifuged.

Single carbon bond, a chemical bond in which two carbon atoms share one electron

Soft drinks, (also called soda drinks or pop) that contain high amounts of sugar

Sprue, severe allergy to the protein gluten that causes inflammation of the small intestines and leads to maldigestion and weight loss

Statins, new drugs which inhibit the synthesis of cholesterol and lower cholesterol levels in the blood

Steatorrhea, excess fat in the stools caused by maldigestion and malabsorption of dietary fat

Sterol regulatory element binding proteins (SREBPs) proteins that bind to and regulate the activity of the SREs/

Sterol regulatory elements (SREs) small gene segments near promoter regions of DNA that regulate the activity of the genes which code for proteins

Thrombin, an enzyme which converts fibrinogen to fibrin that forms a clot

Thrombosis, clots formed in blood or in arteries from aggregation of blood platelets

Thromboxane, a prostaglandin which increases platelet aggregation

Thymine, nitrogen containing organic cyclic compound that is a component of DNA

Thyroxine, a hormone produce by the thyroid gland that regulates the utilization of oxygen in the burning of foods in mitochondria

Tissue plasminogen activator (TPA), a protein which activates plasminogen and forms plasmin

Transcription, the synthesis of mRNA from DNA in which the genetic information in DNA is transcribed to mRNA

Translation, The synthesis of proteins by mRNA in which the genetic information in mRNA is converted to the sequence of the amino acids in the protein.

Tricarboxylic cycle, a series of enzyme reactions in the mitochondria in which acetyl-CoA is oxidized to produce carbon dioxide and water and releases energy

Triglycerides, molecules in which glycerol has three fatty acids attached by ester bonds

Uracil, nitrogen containing cyclic organic compound that occurs in RNA

References

Introduction: General Concepts of Biochemistry and Types of Lipids.

Murray et al. 1988. Harper"s Biochemistry. Twenty first edition. Appleton Lange Pub. Norwalk, Connecticut. There are many introductory books on Biochemistry that will suffice. I recommend this one or a later edition.

Chapter 1 Digestion of Foods, Obesity and the Metabolic Syndrome

Borgstrom, B., Erlanson-Albertsson, C., and Wieloch, T., 1979. Pancreatic colipase chemistry and physiology, J. Lipid Res. 20:805.

Brash, A. 1999. Lipoxygenases: occurrence, functions, catalysis, and acquisition of substrate. J. Biol. Chem., 274: 3679.

Chen, Guoxun, et al., 1996. Disappearance of body fat in normal rats induced by adenovirus-mediated leptin gene therapy. Proc, Natl. Acad. Sci, USA, 93:14799.

Feuerstein, G., and Hallenbech, J.M., 1987. Leukotrienes in health and disease, Fed. Proc. 1:186.

Gainsford, T. et al. 1996. Leptin can induce proliferation differentiation, and functional activation of hemopoietic cells. Proc. Natl. Acad. Sci. USA 93:14568.

Green, P. H. R., and Blackman, R. M., 1981. Intestinal Lipoprotein Metabolism, J. Lipid Res., 22:1153.

Hofmann, A.F., 1970. Gastroenterology: physical events in lipid digestion and absorption, Fed. Proc., 29:1317.

Holm, C. et al. 1988. Hormone-sensitive lipase: sequence, expression, and chromosomal location to 19 cent-q 13.3. Science 241:1503.

Gainsford, T. et al. 1996. Leptin can induce proliferation, differentiation, and functional activation of hemopoietic cells. Proc. Natl. Acad. Sci, USA, 93:14564–14568.

Murray, R. K. et al. 1988. Harper's Biochemistry 21st ed. Appleton Lange, Norwalk, Connecticut.

Matthias T, Smiley D. L,. Heiman, S. and Heiman, M., 2000. Ghrelin induces adiposity in rodents. Nature 407: 908

Muzzin, P. Eisensmith, R. C. Copeland, K. C., and Woo, S. L. C., 1996, Correction of obesity and diabetes in genetically obese mice by leptin gene therapy. Proc. Natl. Acad. Sci. USA 93:14804.

National Institutes of Health, 1998. Clinical guidelines on the identification, evaluation, and treatment of overweight and obesity in adults. Bethesda, Maryland: Department of Health and Human Services, National Institutes of Health, National Heart, Lung, and Blood Institute.

National Research Council. 1989. Diet and health: implications for reducing chronic disease risk. Washington, DC: National Academy Press.

Patton, J.S. and Hofmann, A. F. 1986. Lipid Digestion, Unit 19. in The UndergraduateTeaching Project in Gastroenterology, Liver Disease. American Gastroenterological Association, Milner-Fenwick, Inc, (distrubtor), Timonium, Maryland, p. 14–15, 45–47

Samuelsson, B., Dahlen, S., Lindgren, J.A., Rouzer, C.A., and Serhan, C.N., 1987. Leukotrienes and lipoxins: structures, biosynthesis, and biological effects. Science, 237:171.

Stunkard AJ, Wadden TA. 1993 Eds., Obesity: theory and therapy. Second Edition. NewYork Raven Press.

Wren, A. M. et al. 2000. The novel hypothalamic peptide ghrelin stimulates food intake and growth hormone secretion. Endocrinology 141: 4325–4328.

Chapter 2 Dietary Therapy for High Levels Of Blood Lipids

Anderson, J. W,. et al., 1988. Cholesterol-lowering effects of psyllium hydrophilic mucilloid for hypercholesterolemic men. Arch. Intern. Med. 148:292.

Balasubramaniam, S., Simons, L. A., Chang, S., and Hinkle, J. B., 1985. Reduction in plasma cholesterol and increase in biliary cholesterol by a diet rich in n-3 fatty acids in the rat. J. Lipid Res. 26:684.

Bang, H. O., Dyerberg, J., and Sinclair, H. M., 1980. The composition of the Eskimo food in northwestern Greenland. Am. J. Clin. Nutr. 33:2657.

Barlow, S. M., and Stansby, M. E. eds., 1982. Nutritional Evaluation of Long Chain Fatty Acids in Fish Oil. Academic Press, New York.

Bing, R.J., 1982. Effect of alcohol on the heart and cardiac metabolism. Fed. Proc. 41:2443.

Black, K. L., Culp, B., Madison, D., Randall, O. S., and Lands, W. E. M., 1979, The protective effects on dietary fish oil on focal cerebral infarction. Prostagl. Med., 5:247.

Cohen, L. A., 1987. Diet and cancer, Sci. Am., 257:42.

Connor, W. E., Neuringer, M., and Reisbick, S., 1992. Essential fatty acids: the importance of n-3 content in the retina and brain. Nutr. Rev. 50: 21.

Crouse, J. R., and Grundy, S. M., 1984. Effects of alcohol on plasma lipo-proteins and cholesterol and triglyceride metabolism in man. J. Lipid Res. 25:486.

Dyerberg, J., 1986. Linolenate derived polyunsaturated fatty acids and prevention of atherosclerosis. Nutr. Rev. 44:125.

Dyerberg, J., and Bang, H. O., 1979. Haemostatic function and platelet polyunsaturated fatty acids in Eskimos. Lancet 2:433.

Ehsani, A. A., 1987. Cardiovascular adaptations to exercise training in the elderly. Fed. Proc. 46:1840.

Gerstenblith, G., Renlund, D. G., and Lakatta, E. G., 1987. Cardiovascular response to exercise in younger and older men. Fed. Proc. 46:1834.

Giovannucci, E. et al., 1998. Multivitamin use, folate, and colon cancer in women in the Nurses Health Study. Ann. Intern. Med. 129:517.

Goodnight, S. H., Harris, W. S., Connor, W. E., and Illingworth, D. R., 1982. Polyunsaturated fatty acids, hyperlipidemia and thrombosis. Atheroscl. 2: 87.

Grundy, S. M., 1986. Comparison of monounsaturated fatty acids and carbo-hydrates for lowering plasma cholesterol. N. Engl. J. Med. 314:745.

Hagen. T. M., Liu, et al, 2002. Feeding acetyl-L-carnitine and lipoic acid to old rats significantly improves metabolic function while decreasing oxidative stress. Proc. Natl. Acad. Sci. USA 99:1870–1875.

Hansen, W. S., 1986. The essential nature of linoleic acid in mammals. Trends Biochem. Sci., 11:263.

Harris, S. H., 1989. Fish oils and plasma lipid and lipoprotein metabolism in humans: a critical review. J. Lipid Res. 30:785.

Hartz, A. J., et al. 1984. The association of smoking with cardiomyopathy. N. Engl. J. Med. 311:1201.

Horrocks, L. H., and Yeo, Y. E., 1999. Health benefits of docosahexaenoic acid (DHA). Pharmacologic Research 40: 211.

Hu, F. B., et al., 1997. Dietary fat intake and the risk of coronary heart disease in women. N. Engl. J. Med. 337: 1491.

Hulley, S. B. and Dzvonik, M. L., 1984. Alcohol intake, blood lipids and mortality from coronary heart disease. Clin Nutr. 3:139.

Influence of eggs on plasma lipoproteins. 1985. Nutr. Rev. 43: 263.

Jump. D., 2001, The Biochemistry of n-3 polyunsaturated fatty acids, J. Biol. Chem. 277:8755.

Kritchevsky, D., 1982. Trans fatty acid effects in experimental atherosclerosis. Fed. Proc., 41:2813.

Kromhout, D., Bosschieter, E. B., and De Lezenne Coulander, C., 1985. The inverse relation between fish consumption and 20-year mortality from coronary heart disease. N. Engl. J. Med. 312: 1205.

Lecos, C., 1983, A compendium on fats, FDA Consumer, March.

Lemley, B., What Does Science Say You Should Eat? Discover Magazine, Feb. 2004, pp. 43–49.

Liu, J., Killilea, D. and Ames, B. N., 2002. Age-associated mitochondrial oxidative decay:Improvement carnitine acetyltransferase substrate binding affinity and activity in brain by feeding old rats acetyl-L-carnitine and/or R-α-lipoic acid. Proc. Natl. Acad. Sci. USA, 99:1876–1881.

Marinetti, G.V. 1990. Disorders of Lipid Metabolism. Plenum Press, New York.

Marnett, L.J., et al., 1999. Arachidonic acid oxygenation by COX-1 and COX-2. J. Biol. Chem. 274, 22903

Marcus, A. J., 1984. The eicosanoids in biology and medicine. J. Lipid Res., 25:1511.

Mattson, F. H., and Grundy, S. M., 1985. Comparison of effects of dietary saturated, monounsaturated, and polyunsaturated fatty acids on plasma lipids and lipoproteins in man, J. Lipid Res. 26:194.

Mertz, W., 1982. Trace minerals and atherosclerosis. Fed. Proc. 41:2807.

Mezey, E., 1985. Metabolic effects of alcohol, Fed. Proc. 44:134.

Miller, R. W., 1986. Diet, exercise, and other keys to a healthy heart, FDA Consumer, February issue.

Moderate alcohol consumption increases plasma high density lipoprotein cholesterol, 1987. Nutr. Rev. 45:8.

National Cholesterol Education Program Expert Panel, 1988. Report of the National Cholesterol Education Expert Panel on detection, evaluation, and treatment of high blood cholesterol in adults. Arch. Intern. Med., 148:360.

Nettleton, J. A., 1985. Seafood Nutrition. Facts, Issues, and Marketing of Nutrition in Fish and Shellfish. Osprey Books, Huntington, New York.

Normand, F., 1987. Binding of bile acids and trace minerals by soluble hemicellulose of rice. Food Technol. 41:87.

Pariza, M. W., 1987. Dietary fat, calorie restriction, ad libitum feeding, and cancer risk. Nutr. Rev., 45:1.

Phillipson, B. E., et al., 1985. Reduction of plasma lipids, lipoproteins, and apoproteins by dietary fish oils in patients with hypertriglyceridemia. N. Engl. J. Med. 312:1210.

Shigenaga, M. K., Hagen, T. M., and Ames, B. N., 1994. Oxidative damage and mitochondrial decay in aging. Proc. Natl. Acad. Sci., USA, 95:10771–10778.

Sirtori, C., Rucci, G., and Gorini, S. eds. 1975. Diet and Atherosclerosis. Plenum Press, New York.

Slavin, J. L., 1987. Dietary fiber: classification, chemical analysis, and food sources. J. Am. Dietetic Assoc. 87:1164.

Vahouny, G. V., 1982. Dietary fiber, lipid metabolism, and atherosclerosis. Fed. Proc., 41:2801.

Van Horn, L., et al., 1988. Serum lipid responses to a fat-modified oatmeal-enhanced diet. Prev. Med. 17:377.

Willis, A. L., 1981. Nutritional and pharmacological factors in eicosanoid biology. Nutr. Rev. 39:289.

Willett, W., C., and Skerritt, J., 2005. Eat drink and be healthy. Co-Developed with the Harvard School of Public Health. Pub.

Willett, W. C., Dietz, W. H., and Colditz, G. A., 1999. Guidelines for healthy weight. N. Engl. J. Med. 341:427.

Wood, P. D., Terry, R. B., and Haskell, W. L., 1985. Metabolism of substrates: diet, lipoprotein metabolism and exercise. Fed. Proc. 44:358.

Zanni, E. E., et al., 1987. Effect of egg cholesterol and dietary fats on plasma lipids, lipoproteins, and apoproteins of normal women consuming natural diets. J. Lipid Res. 28:518.

Chapter 3 Drug Therapies For High Levels Of Blood Lipids And The Treatment Of Blood Clots

Benditt, E. P., and Schwarz, S. M., 1984. Atherosclerosis: what can we learn from studies in human tissues. Lab. Invest. 50:3.

Blankenhorn, D. H., et al., 1987. Beneficial effects of combined colestipol-niacin therapy on coronary atherosclerosis and coronary venous bypass grafts. J. Am. Med. Assoc. 257:3233.

Brown, M. S. and Goldstein, J. L. 1986. A receptor-mediated pathway for cholesterol homeostasis. Science 232:34.

Canner, P. L. et al., 1986. Fifteen year mortality in coronary drug project patients: long-term benefit with niacin. J. Am. Coll. Cardiol. 8:1245.

Castelli, W. P. et al., 1986. Incidence of coronary heart disease and lipoprotein cholesterol levels, the Framingham study. J. Am. Med. Assoc., 256:2835.

Chesebro, J. H., et al., 1984. Effect of dipyridamole and aspirin on late vein-graft patency after coronary bypass operations. N. Engl. J. Med., 310:209.

Consensus conference, 1985. Lowering blood cholesterol to prevent heart disease. J. Am. Med. Assoc. 253:2080.

East, C., Grundy, S. M., and Bilheimer, D. W., 1986. Normal cholesterol levels with lovastatin (mevinolin) therapy in a child with homozygous familial hypercholesterolemia following liver transplantation. J. Am. Med. Assoc. 256:2843.

Expert Panel, 1988. Report of the National Cholesterol Education Program Expert Panel on detection, evaluation, and treatment of high blood cholesterol in adults. Arch. Inter. Med. 148:36.

Goldberg, R. J., Gore, J. M., Dalen J. E., and Alpert, J. S., 1986. Long-term anticoagulant therapy after acute myocardial infarction. Am. Heart J. 109:616.

Grundy, S. M., 1986, Cholesterol and coronary heart disease. A new era, J. Am. Med. Assoc., 256:2849.

Huddleston, C. B., et al., Amelioration of the deleterious effects of platelets activated during cardiopulmonary bypass: comparison of a thromboxane synthetase inhibitor and a prostacyclin analogue. J. Thorac, Cardiovasc. Surg, 89:190.

Jonasson, L., Bondjers, G., and Hansson, G. K., 1987. Lipoprotein lipase in atherosclerosis: its presence in smooth muscle cells and absence from macrophages. J. Lipid Res. 28:437.

Kinosian, B. P., and Eisenberg, J. M., 1988. Cutting into cholesterol: cost-effective alternatives for treating hypercholesterolemia. J. Am. Med. Assoc. 259:2249.

Kuo, P. T. et al., 1981. Familial type II hyperlipoproteinemia with coronary heart disease. Effect of diet, colestipol, and nicotinic acid treatment, Chest 79:286.

Marinetti, G.V. 1990. Disorders of Lipid Metabolism. Plenum Press, New York.

Pedersen, A. K., and Fitzgerald, G. A., 1984. Dose-related kinetics of aspirin: presystemic acetylation of platelet cyclooxygenase. N. Engl. J. Med. 311:1206.

Rapp, J. H., Connor, E. E., Lin, D. S., Inahara, T., and Porter, J. M., 1983. Lipids of human atherosclerotic plaques and xanthomas: clues to the mechanism of plaque formation. J. Lipid Res. 24:1329.

Roberts, A. B., et al., 1983. Selective accumulation of low density lipoproteins on damaged arterial wall. J. Lipid Res. 24:1160.

Ross, R., and Glomset, J. A., 1976. The pathogenesis of atherosclerosis. N. Engl. J. Med. 295:369.

Rudel, L. L., et al., 1986. Low density lipoproteins in atherosclerosis, J. Lipid Res., 27:465.

Rundek, T. 2004. Atorvastatin decreases the CoQ10 level in the blood of patients at risk for cardiovascular disease and stroke. Arch. Neurol. 61:889

Scanu, A. M., Wissler, R. W., and Getz, G. S. eds, 1979, The Biochemistry of Atherosclerosis. Marcel Dekker, New York.

Shepherd, J. 1980, Cholestyramine promotes receptor-mediated low-density-lipoprotein catabolism, N. Engl. J. Med., 301:1219.

Stamler, J., Wentworth, D., and Neaton, J. D., 1986. MRFIT Research Group, Is relationship between serum cholesterol and risk of premature death from coronary heart disease continuous and graded? Findings in 356,222 primary screens of the MRFIT, J. Am. Med. Assoc. 256:2823.

Starzi, T. E., et al., 1984. Heart-liver transplantation in a patient with familial hypercholesterolemia. Lancet i:1382.

Strong, J. P., 1986, Coronary atherosclerosis in soldiers. A clue to the natural history of atherosclerosis in the young. J. Am. Med. Assoc. 256:2863.

The lipid research clinics coronary primary prevention trial results. 1984. Reduction in incidence of coronary heart disease. J. Am. Med. Assoc. 251:351.

Chapter 4 Atherosclerosis and Coronary Artery Disease (CAD).

Anderson, K. M., Castelli, W. P., and Levy, D., 1987. Cholesterol and mortality: 30 years of follow-up from the Framingham study. J. Am. Med. Assoc. 257:2176.

Benditt, E. P., and Schwarz, S. M., 1984. Atherosclerosis: what can we learn from studies in human tissues. Lab. Invest. 50:3.

Brown, M. S., and Goldstein, J. L., 1984 How LDL receptors influence cholesterol and atherosclerosis. Sci. Amer., 251:58.

Brown, M. S. and Goldstein, J. J., 1986. A receptor-mediated pathway for cholesterol homeostasis. Science 232:34.

Castelli, W. P., 1986. The triglyceride issue: a view from Framingham, Am. Heart J., 112:432.

Chisolm G. M. Hazen, S. L., Fox, P. L., and Cathcart, M. K., 1999. The oxidation of lipoproteins by monocytes-macrophages. J. Biol. Chem. 274:25959.

Castelli, W. P., et al. 1986. Incidence of coronary heart disease and lipoprotein cholesterol levels: the Framingham study. J. Am. Med. Assoc. 256:2835.

Curtiss, L. K., Black, A. S., Takagi, Y., and Plow, E. F., 1987. New mechanism for foam cell generation in atherosclerotic lesions. J. Clin. Invest. 86:367.

Desai, K., Bruckdorfer, K. R., Hutton, R. A., and Owen, J. S., 1989. Binding of apoE-rich high density lipoprotein particles by saturable sites on human blood platelets inhibits agonist-induced platelet aggregation. J. Lipid Res., 30:831.

Etingin, O. R., Weksler, B. B., and Hajjar, D. P., 1986. Cholesterol metabolism is altered by hydrolytic metabolites of prostacyclin in arterial smooth muscle cells. J. Lipid Res., 27:530.

Expert panel, 1988, Report of the national cholesterol education program expert panel on detection, evaluation, and treatment of high blood cholesterol in adults, Arch. Intern. Med., 148:36.

Goldbourt, U., Holtzman, E., and Neufeld, H. N., 1985. Total and high density lipoprotein cholesterol in the serum and risk of mortality: evidence of a threshold effect. Brit. Med. J., 290:1239.

Grundy, S.M., 1986. Cholesterol and coronary heart disease. J. Am. Med. Assoc. 256:2849.

Grundy, S. M., 1986. Cholesterol and coronary heart disease: a new era. J. Am. Med. Assoc. 256:2849.

Harlan, J. M., and Haker, L. A., 1983. Thrombosis and Coronary Artery Disease. Upjohn Co., Kalamazoo, Michigan.

Hegele, R. A., et al. 1986. Aplipoprotein B-gene DNA polymorphisms associated with myocardial infarction. N. Engl. J. Med. 315:1509.

Kannel, W. B., 1983. High-density lipoproteins: epidemiologic profile and risks of coronary artery disease. Am. J. Cardiol. 52:9B

Kher, N. and Marsh, J.D., 2004. Pathobiology of Atherosclerosis: Seminars in Thrombosis and Hemostasis. 30: 665–672.

Kromhout, D., Bosscheiter, E. B., and De Lezenne Coulander, C., 1985. The inverse relation between fish consumption and 20-year mortality from coronary heart disease. N. Engl. J. Med. 312:1205.

Kuo, P. T, Kostis, J. B., Moreyra, A. E., and Hayes, J. A., 1981. Familial type II hyperlipoproteinemia with coronary heart disease. Effect of diet-colestipol-nicotinic acid treatment. Chest. 79: 286.

Marinetti, G.V. 1990. Disorders of Lipid Metabolism. Plenum Press, New York.

Multiple risk factor intervention trial research group: multiple risk factor intervention trial. Risk factor changes and mortality results, 1982. J. Am. Med. Assoc. 248:1465.

Nagy, L., Tontonoz, P., Alvarez, J.G.A., Chen, H., and Evans, R.M., 1998. Oxidized LDL regulates macrophage gene expression through ligand activation of PPAR-γ. Cell 93:229–240

Olson, R. E., 1986 Mass intervention vs. screening and selective intervention for the prevention of coronary heart disease. J. Am. Med. Assoc. 255:2204.

Pooling project research group. Relationship of blood pressure, serum cholesterol, relative weight, and ECG abnormalities to incidence of major coronary events: final report of the Pooling Project. 1978, J. Chron. Dis. 31:201.

Paoletti, R., Gotto, A. M. Jr., and Hajjar, D. P., 2004. Inflammation in atherosclerosis and implications for therapy. Circulation 109:20–26.

Roberts, A. B., et al., 1983. Selective accumulation of low density lipoproteins on damaged arterial wall. J. Lipid Res. 24:1160.

Ross, R., and Glomset, J. A., 1976. The pathogenesis of atherosclerosis. N. Engl. J. Med., 295:369.

Rudel, L. L., Parks, J. S., Johnson, F. L., and Babiak, J., 1986. Low density lipoproteins in atherosclerosis. J. Lipid Res. 27: 465.

Scanu, A. M., Wissler, R. W., and Getz, G. S. (eds.), 1979. The Biochemistry of Atherosclerosis. Marcel Dekker, New York.

Siegel, D., Grady, D., Browner, W. S., and Hulley, S. B., 1988. Risk factor modification after myocardial infarction. Ann. Intern. Med. 108:213.

Stamler, J., Wentworth, D., and Neaton, J. D., 1986. MRFIT Research Group, is relationship between serum cholesterol and risk of premature death from coronary heart disease continuous and graded? Findings in 356,222 primary screens of the MRFIT, J. Am. Med. Assoc. 256:2823.

Starzi, T.E., et al., 1984, Heart-liver transplantation in a patient with familial hypercholesterolemia, Lancet, i:1382.

Steinberg, D. 1997. Low Density Lipoprotein Oxidation and Its Pathological Significance. J. Biol. Chem. 272: 20963–20966.

Strong, J. P., 1986. Coronary Atherosclerosis in Soldiers. A clue to the natural history of atherosclerosis in the young. J. Am. Med. Assoc., 256:2863.

Wynder, E. L., Field, F., and Haley, N. J., 1986. Population screening for cholesterol determination, a pilot study. J. Am. Med. Assoc. 256:2839.

Chapter 5 Metabolism of Fatty Acids

Borum, R. 1981. Possible carnitine requirement of the newborn and the effect of genetic disease on the carnitine requirement. Nutrition. Rev. 39:385.

Brash, A, 1999, Lipoxygenases, occurrence, functions, catalysis, and acquisition of substrate. J. Biol. Chem., 274: 3679.

Carnitine metabolism in man, 1980. Nutr. Rev. 38:338.

Duplus, E., Glorian, M., Forest, C. 2000. Fatty acid regulation of gene transcription. J. Biol. Chem., 275, 30749.

Engel, A. G., and Angelini, C., 1973. Carnitine deficiency of human skeletal muscle with associated lipid storage myopathy: a new syndrome. Science. 179:899.

Jump. D., 2001. The Biochemistry of n-3 polyunsaturated fatty acids. J. Biol. Chem. 277:8755.

Marnett, L.J. Rowlinson, S. W., Goodwin, D.C, Kalgutkar, A. S. and Lanzo, C. A., 1999. Arachidonic acid oxygenation by COX-1 and COX-2. J. Biol. Chem. 274, 22903

Marinetti, G. V., 1990. Disorders of Lipid Metabolism. Plenum Press, New York.

Murray, R. K., Granner, D. K., Mayes, P. A., and Rodwell, V. W. 1988. Harper's Biochemistry. 21st ed., Appleton Lange, Publ. Norwalk, Connecticut.

Neuringer, M., and Connor, W. E., 1986. Omega-3 fatty acids in the brain and retina: evidence for their essentiality. Nutr. Rev. 44:285.

Press, M, Kikuchi, H., Shimoyama, T., and Thompson, G. R., 1974. Diagnosis and treatment of essential fatty acid deficiency in man. Brit. Med. J. 2:247.

Stryer, L., 1988. Biochemistry, 3rd ed., W. H. Freeman Co., San Francisco.

Systemic carnitine deficiency. 1981. Nutr. Rev. 39:400.

Chapter 6 Cholesterol Metabolism and Bile Acids

Carey, M., C., 1978. Critical tables for calculating cholesterol saturation in bile. J. Lipid Res., 19:945.

Duncan, E. A., Brown, M. S., Goldstein, J. L., and Sakai, J., 1997. Cleavage site for sterol-regulated protease localized to a leu-ser bond in the luminal loop of the sterol regulatory element binding protein-2. J. Biol. Chem. 272:12778.

Marinetti, G. V., 1990. Disorders of Lipid Metabolism. Plenum Press, New York.

Murray, R. K., Granner, D. K., Mayes, P. A., and Rodwell, V. W., 1988. Harper's Biochemistry, 21st ed., Appleton Lange, Norwalk, Connecticut.

Sabine, J., R., 1977. Cholesterol. Marcel Dekker, New York.

Chapter 7 Metabolism of Blood Lipoproteins.

Aviram, M., Bierman, E. L., and Oram, J. F., 1989. High density lipoprotein stimulates sterol translocation between intracellular and plasma membrane pools in human monocyte-derived macrophages, J. Lipid Res. 30:65.

Beaumont, J. L., Carlson, L. A., Cooper, G. R., Fejar, Z., and Fredrickson, D. S., 1970. Classification of hyperlipidaemias and hyperlipoproteinemias. Bull WHO 43:1970

Bondy, P. K., and Rosenberg, L. E. 1980. Metabolic Control and Disease. 8th ed., W. B. Saunders Co., Philadelphia.

Brenninkmeijer, B. J., Stuyt, P. M. J., Demacker, P. N. M., Stalenhoef, A. F. H. and van't Laar, A., 1987. Catabolism of chylomicron remnants in normolipid-emic subjects in relation to the apoprotein E phenotype. J. Lipid Res. 28:361.

Breslow, J. L., 1987. Genetic regulation of apolipoproteins, Am. Heart J. 113:422.

Brown, M. S., and Goldstein, J. L., 1984. How LDL receptors influence cho-lesterol and atherosclerosis, Sci. Amer. 251:58.

Brown, M. S. and Goldstein, J. L. 1986. A receptor-mediated pathway for cho-lesterol homeostasis. Science, 232:34.

Capurso, A., et al. 1988. Apolipoprotein C-II deficiency: detection of immuno-reactive apolipoprotein C-II in the intestinal mucosa of two patients. J. Lipid Res. 29:703.

Curtiss, L. K., Black, A. S., Takagi, Y., and Plow, E. F., 1987. New mechanism for foam cell generation in atherosclerotic lesions, J. Clin. Invest. 86:367.

Duncan, E. A., Brown, M. S, Goldstein, J. L., and Sakai, J., 1997. Cleavage site for sterol-regulated protease localized to a leu-ser bond in the luminal loop of the sterol regulatory element binding protein-2. J. Biol. Chem. 272:12778.

Gerrity, R. G., 1981. The role of the monocyte in atherogenesis. I. Transition of blood-borne monocytes into foam cells in fatty lesions. Am. J. Pathol. 103:181.

Ghiselli, G., Schaefer, E. J., Gascon, P., and Brewer, H. B. Jr., 1981. Type III hyperlipoproteinemia with apolipoprotein E deficiency. Science 214:1239.

Goldstein, J. L., and Brown, M. S., 1984. Progress in understanding the LDL receptor and HMG-CoA reductase, two membrane proteins that regulate plasma cholesterol. J. Lipid Res. 25:1450.

Goldstein, J. L. Kita, T. and Brown, M. S. 1983. Defective lipoprotein recep-tors and atherosclerosis. N. Engl. J. Med. 309:288.

Grundy, S.M., 1984. Pathogenesis of hyperlipoproteinemia. J. Lipid Res. 25:1611.

Heart-liver transplantation in a child with homozygous familial hypercholes-terolemia. 1985. Nutr. Rev., 43:274.

Hoeg, J. M., Gregg, R. E., and Brewer, H. B., 1986. An approach to the management of hyperlipoproteinemia. J. Am. Med. Assoc., 255:512.

Howard, B. V., 1987. Lipoprotein metabolism in diabetes mellitus. J. Lipid Res. 28:613.

Jonasson, L., Bondjers, G., and Hansson, G. K., 1987. Lipoprotein lipase in atherosclerosisits presence in smooth muscle cells and absence from macrophages. J. Lipid Res. 28:437.

Kuusi, T., Taskinen, M. R., Solakivi, T., and Makelin, R. K., 1988. Role of apolipoproteins E and C in type V hyperlipoproteinemia, J. Lipid Res. 29:293.

Lusis, A. J., 1988. Genetic factors affecting blood lipoproteins: the candidate gene approach. J. Lipid Res. 29:397.

Mahley, R. W., 1988. Apolipoprotein E: cholesterol transport protein with expanding role in cell biology. Science 240:622.

Mahley, R. W., et al. 1984. Plasma lipoproteins: apoprotein structure and function. J. Lipid Res. 25:1277.

Marinetti, G. V., 1990. Disorders of Lipid Metabolism. Plenum Press, New York.

Naito, H. K., 1988. Apolipoproteins as biochemical markers of cardiac risk. Am. Clin. Lab. January 1988, table 2, p. 28.

Ordovas, J. M., et al., 1987. Apolipoprotein E isoform phenotypic methodology and population frequency with identification of ApoE1 and ApoE5 isoforms. J. Lipid Res. 28:371.

Sprecher, D. L., et al. 1988. Identification of an apoC-II variant (apoC-IIBethesda) in a kindred with apoC-II deficiency and type I hyperlipoproteinemia. J. Lipid Res. 29:273.

Sudhof, T. C., Goldstein, J. L., Brown, M. S., and Russell, D. W., 1985. The LDL receptor gene: a mosaic of exons shared with different proteins. Science 228:815.

Tall, A. R., 1986. Plasma lipid transfer proteins. J. Lipid Res. 27:361.

The lipid research clinics coronary primary prevention trial results, reduction in incidence of coronary heart disease, II. The relationship of reduction in incidence of coronary heart disease to cholesterol lowering. 1984. J. Am. Med. Assoc., 251:351.

Walton, K. W. 1975. Pathogenic mechanisms in atherosclerosis. Am. J. Cardiol., 35:542.

Zilversmit, D. B., 1973. A proposal linking atherogenesis to the interaction of endothelial lipoprotein lipase with triglyceride-rich lipoproteins. Circul. 33:633.

Chapter 8 Excess Dietary Carbohydrates are Converted To Fat And Cause Obesity.

Duncan, E. A., Brown, M. S. Goldstein, J.L. and Sakai, J. 1997. Cleavage site for sterol-regulated protease localized to a leu-ser bond in the luminal loop of the sterol regulatory element binding protein-2. J. Biol. Chem. 272:12778.

Duplus, E., Glorian, M., Forest, C. 2000. Fatty acid regulation of gene transcription. J. Biol. Chem., 275, 30749.

Olefsky, J.M, 1999. Insulin stimulated glucose transport. J. Biol. Chem. 274:1863.

Osborne, T.F., 2000. Sterol regulatory element-binding proteins (SREBPs). Key regulators of nutritional homeostasis and insulin action. J. Biol. Chem. 275: 32379.

Appendix

Information on conversions of weights and measures

1 kg = 2.2 lbs.

70 kg = 154.3 lbs

1 oz = 29.57 ml

1 glass = 8 oz

1 teaspoon = 15 ml

1 inch = 2.54 cm

1 foot = 30.48 cm

1 yard = 91/44 cm

1 mile = 1669.3 m

1 km = 1093.6 yards

F = 9/5(C) + 42 degrees

C = 5/9 (F-32) degrees

100 F = 37.8 C degrees

98.6 F = 37.0 C degrees

1 grain = 60 mg

Normal ranges for blood chemistry tests (vary from different laboratories)

Sodium   132–146 mmol/L

Potassium   3.5–5.5 mmol/L

Chloride   92–109 mmol/L

Bicarbonate   24–31 mmol/L

Glucose   70–110 mg/dL (taken on fasting blood sample)

BUN   8–25 mg/dL BUN, blood urea nitrogen, comes from the break-down of proteins

Creatinine   0.5–1.5 mg/dL Creatinine comes from the breakdown of creatine in muscles

BUN and creatinine levels indicate how well the kidneys are working

Calcium ions 4.25–5.25 mg/dL

Magnesium   1.6–3.0 mg/dL

Phosphorus   2.6–4.6 mg/dL

Uric acid   2.4–7.5 mg/dL, uric acid comes from the breakdown of nucleotides and is high in persons with gout

Total protein 5.7–8.2 g/dL

Albumin, 3.2–4.8 g/dL

Enzyme tests for liver function:

Alk, 45–129 U/L (alkaline phosphatase)

SGOT, AST, 0–34 U/L. (SGOT =aspartate aminotransaminase

SGPT, ALT, 12–49 U/L (SGPT = alanine aminotransaminase

LDH, 50–240 U/L (LDH=lactate dehydrogenase)

CPK, 5–200 U/L CPK=creatinine-phosphokinase

Tests for cancer

CEA, 0–2.5 ng/ml, carcinoma embryonic antigen

PSA, 0–4.0 ng/ml. (PSA, prostate specific antigen)

Blood lipid analyses

Cholesterol (total), < 200 mg/dl

LDL cholesterol, < 100 mg/dL (LDL, low density lipoprotein)

HDL cholesterol, 40–45 mg/dL for men, (HDL, high density lipoprotein)

HDL cholesterol, 50–75 mg/dL for women

Triglycerides, 30–150 mg/dl (some labs use <130 mg/dl)

Pancreatic enzymes

Amylase, 60–180 U/L

Lipase, 4–25 U/L

Prostate tests for men

PSA, 0–4.0 ng/ml (PSA, prostate specific antigen)

Acid phosphatase, total, 0–10 U/L

Acid phosphatase, < 4 U/L

Test for anemia

Iron, 60–170 μg/dl

TIBC, 240–425 μg/dl (TIBC, total iron binding capacity)

Ferritin, 22–320 ng/ml (ferritin is a protein that contains stored iron)

Transferrin, 220–730 picograms/ml (transferring transports iron through the blood to the liver)

Transferrin saturated, 20–255%

Other tests include erythropoietin, a protein which stimulates the synthesis of red and white blood cells in bone marrow, Vit.B-12, and or Vit.B-12 intrinsic factor that is made in the stomach and allows vitamin B-12 to be absorbed into the blood. A deficieny of vitamin B-12 intrinsic factor causes pernicious anemia.

Hemotology tests

Hb, Hemoglobin, Males 14–18 g/dL

Hb for women, 12–16 g/dL

Hct=Hematocrit, M 40–52 %, (hematocrit is the percent of spun blood which are red cells

Hct=Hematocrit, F 37–52 %

RBC, Men, 4.6–6.2 million/microliter (RBC, red blood cell count)

RBC, women, 4.1–5.5 million/microliter

MCV, M 80–90 fL (fL=femtoliter)

MCV, F 80–96 fL MCV, mean corpuscular (red cell) volume)

WBC, 5000–10000/µL (WBC, white cell blood cell count)

Platelets, 150,000–400,000/µL

Bleeding time, < 5–6 minutes by the Ivy test (time to clot after a small incision made on the skin)

Thrombin time, 10–14 seconds (time to form a clot after the enzyme thombin is added to a sample of plasma)

Fibrinogen, 200–400 mg/dL

Blood pH (acidity), 7.35–7.45 (slightly alkaline since in the pH scale 7.0 is neutral, above 7.0 is alkaline and below 7.0 is acidic

Endocrinology

Thyroxine T4   5.0–12 µg/dL (done by radioimmunoassay)

T4 Thyroxine, free   0.8–2.2 ng/dl

Thyroxine T3,   75–200 ng/dl

TSH, 0.27–4. µU/ml (TSH =thyroid stimulating hormone)

Aldostrone, 3–12 ng/ml supine and 5–25 ng/ml upright

Growth hormone, 1–10 ng/ml

About the Author

Guido V. Marinetti has a Ph.D. degree in Biochemistry and is Professor Emeritus at the University of Rochester Medical School. He taught undergraduate, graduate, and medical students biochemistry for 40 years. During this time he did research on developing chromatographic methods for separating and analyzing phospholipids, and studied the arrangement and functions of phospholipids in cell membranes. He taught medical students the hyperlipoproteinemias, cholesterol and heart disease, and how diet and drugs are used to treat patients with high levels of blood lipids.

Marinetti edited a three volume series entitled *Lipid Chromatographic Analysis* (Dekker, 1976) and authored a book entitled *Disorders of Lipid Metabolism* (Plenum, 1990). He also has published many articles in a variety of well-known biochemical journals.

Index

978-0-595-39580-4
0-595-39580-5

www.ingramcontent.com/pod-product-compliance
Lightning Source LLC
Chambersburg PA
CBHW020423290526
45785CB00002B/694

* 9 7 8 0 5 9 5 3 9 5 8 0 4 *